To Barbara
With thanks and love for enduring the
years this book was in the making

For Bryan King

Thanks fo. the honor of

Signing your book

From the Everyday
Everyday
to the Extraordinary

West Virginia Pharmacists' Stories

Douglas
Glover,
R.Ph., M.D.

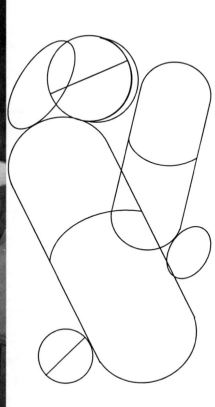

Edited by
Dr. Marie Abate
and
Dr. Arthur Jacknowitz

Table of Contents

Foreword: It's About the People

Dennis B. Worthen, Ph.D.
Lloyd Scholar
Lloyd Library and Museum
Cincinnati, OH

My first contact with Doug Glover was in 1997 when I was researching pharmacists and pharmacy during World War II.[1] He shared the story of his father in northern West Virginia. With a population of 1500, there was only a single pharmacist in Rowlesburg; Glover's Drug Store was a vital part of the community during the war years. Even then Doug Glover grasped that the stories of pharmacy practice and practitioners were important and worth recording. It is no wonder that he finally turned to finding and sharing the West Virginia stories so painstakingly gathered for this book.

George Urdang, pharmacy historian and co-author of Kremers and Urdang's *History of Pharmacy*, wrote in 1950 of the need to capture the development of pharmacy in the states.[2] He noted that one of the few examples up to that date was *The Annals of Pharmacy in West Virginia* by Roy Bird Cook and encouraged more of the same type of work. Since then, a number of works have appeared about Iowa (Lee Anderson), New Jersey (David Cowen), and Arizona (George Bender), among others. There have also been a number of histories about colleges of pharmacy and state associations. Each of these provides an important view of pharmacy and pharmacists.

This book is an ambitious project that tells stories of the men and women in pharmacy rather than just reciting events and happenings. Glover pulls all the threads of the profession together in recounting the stories of West Virginia pharmacists.

The story begins with an overview of the early years and summarizes Cook's 1946 booklet, *The Annals of Pharmacy in West Virginia*. However, Glover does not follow the thematic approach of state board, association, and college used by Cook; instead he focuses on the people. These people range from the founders of what would eventually become Sterling Drug, Inc. and American Home Products, two national manufacturing concerns, to those who served as mayors of West Virginia municipalities both large and small, and state legislators. Leaders in education, politics, and professional associations are all included in five parts and seven appendices of the book.

In *The Annals of Pharmacy in West Virginia,* Cook provided a list of pharmacists and pharmacy students who served in World War I and II. Glover built on the list by providing the details of some of the veterans. Stories of veterans of later conflicts, such as Korea, are also included in the chapter "Behind the Counter to the Front Lines." In an interesting progression, the following chapter recounts the quiet heroism and community service of pharmacists at home during disasters of flood and storm. The latter is a topic frequently mentioned but seldom captured and recorded in a professional history.

The chapters on the West Virginia University School of Pharmacy focus on the deans and emeritus faculty. This excellent approach provides insights into the challenges and accomplishments of educational leaders over the life of the institution. It certainly makes better reading than the dry progression of enrollment and graduation statistics, space and curricula changes, and other institutional data.

The section on professional leadership encompasses the types of materials that one would expect to find in a book of this nature. Chapters on state and national leaders and award winners provide information on individuals and their accomplishments in more detail than just a list of names and places.

Speaker of the U.S. House of Representatives Tip O'Neal commented that "all politics are local" when explaining the impact of the local scene on national politics. The same observation is true in pharmacy: the stories of West Virginia are representative of pharmacy on a national level. It is the pharmacists, on the local level, who were responsible for what happened to the profession. But the work of gathering and sharing those stories is never easy, nor quick, nor straight forward. Doug Glover has succeeded in the task he set out to do – it's about the people.

---

[1] Worthen, D.B. *Pharmacy in World War II,* Binghamton, NY. Haworth Press, 2004

[2] Urdang, G. Forward in Griffenhagen, G.B. *The Story of California Pharmacy,* Madison, WI. American Institute of History of Pharmacy, 1950

Introduction

This book is about pharmacy in West Virginia and the professionals who practice this art. Pharmacists are ubiquitous; they reside in small towns and cities and are a repository of local and regional history. They are leaders of their communities where they have served as mayors and legislators. They have knowledge of their professions' history, an ability to shape its future, and at times they become heroes through no design of their own. This book is about these individuals and how their profession has evolved over the past hundred years.

Before I became an obstetrician and gynecologist, I earned a pharmacy degree from West Virginia University School of Pharmacy and practiced pharmacy for 12 years. Two years ago, after 39 years of delivering babies, I retired. Retirement, which was not to my liking, lasted a month. I was bored and my wife couldn't stand having me under foot. After consulting with Clarke Ridgway and Art Jacknowitz, the co-curators of the Cook-Hayman Pharmacy Museum at the West Virginia University School of Pharmacy, then Dean George Spratto made me an offer I enthusiastically accepted: in return for an office, secretary, computer, and telephone I should write a book about West Virginia pharmacists. But what could I write about and how would I start? I went to see a noted University professor with many books to his credit seeking his advice and guidance. To my chagrin he advised me that very few people would be interested in a book about pharmacists and to forget about the project. With my resolve thus fortified I embarked on this journey.

My interest in this subject was aroused a decade ago by a book I read about the patent medicine business. Emerging from those pages was a tale of two young entrepreneurs with beginnings in the rural West Virginia community of Sistersville, an unlikely point of origin for leading players in our modern pharmaceutical industry. The authors of that book had thoroughly researched one of those youths, but short shrift was given the other. This book, with its many meanderings, is the outcome of my search for the story of the second youth, Albert Diebold.

Stories of events that have shaped West Virginia pharmacy history are the heart and soul of this undertaking. I had not appreciated how resourceful pharmacists are until I began to research this book. When possible, I let them speak for themselves since they experienced the events that form the basis for this work. If available, I used corroborating witnesses to verify statements made. In some cases I spoke from my own knowledge of events.

This work is divided into five parts. The first reviews the early history of the profession in West Virginia, including the story of the young men referred to earlier who began their careers by hawking patent medicines from the back of a horse-drawn buckboard. The second addresses public service by pharmacists beyond their usual duties and responsibilities, whether through public office, the military, or circumstances beyond their control. Part Three chronicles the history of pharmacy education in West Virginia and its advances over the past century. Professional achievements, fulfillment, and recognition are discussed in Part Four, with changing roles and responsibilities reviewed in the last section. The influence pharmacy has had on the history of West Virginia is the story that follows.

Douglas D. Glover, R.Ph., M.D.
Morgantown, West Virginia
October, 2008

Acknowledgements

The greatest pleasure of completing a book is to publicly thank the many people who have both materially and philosophically contributed to its creation. This book opens with a summary of Dr. Roy Bird Cook's magnificent work, *The Annals of Pharmacy in West Virginia*, written in 1943 and published three years later. Dr. Cook chronicles the evolution of the pharmacy profession from colonial days to World War II. An accomplished historian, Dr. Cook's writings serve as a foundation for this book. I am grateful to the West Virginia Pharmacists Association, as owner of the copyright, for supplying the manuscript of Dr. Cook's treatise.

A major debt of gratitude is owed Kate Quinn of Wheeling, WV, who guided my research of entrepreneurs William Weiss and Albert Diebold. Librarians at the Genealogy Division of the Stark County District Library in Canton, Ohio, where Weiss and Diebold were born, provided significant information that contributed to the accuracy of their story. I am grateful to Bill Winsley of The Ohio State Board of Pharmacy for the time he spent checking the accuracy of my statements. Of particular help to me in my research were the Fawcett family (descendents of Albert Diebold), of which Jane and Julie Fawcett and Carol Brown deserve particular praise, as does Louis Bockius III.

A special thank you to Constance Baston, researcher at the Charleston, WV, Veterans Memorial; Debra Basham, archivist at Charleston; John C. Davis, clerk, Census Record, Ancestry Library at Charleston; Bobbie Elliott of Charleston; Brenda Moore, extension librarian of the Fayette County Public Libraries at Oak Hill, WV; Gwen Hubbard, librarian, Brooke County Library at Wellsburg, WV; Peggy Tebbetts, Wheeling-Ohio County genealogist, and Sandy Day, genealogist at the Schiappa Branch of the

Public Library of Steubenville-Jefferson County, Ohio, each of whom were of enormous help with my research. John A. Cuthbert of the West Virginia Collection at the Wise Library of West Virginia University, along with Grace Gmeindl, Steve Shackelford, Jean Siebert and Sally Brown of the WVU Health Sciences Library are likewise truly appreciated. Anita Henry of the Reference Department of the Raleigh County, WV, Public Library was very resourceful and added important information.

Herald M. Forbes, Associate Curator of the West Virginia Regional History Collection of the Wise Library at West Virginia University, made valuable contributions to Chapters 1, 3, 4, 5, and 6 which include supplying Dr. Roy Bird Cook's manuscript, *Alaskan Trophies Won and Lost* (1928), and obituaries of Donald C. Sinclair from the Wheeling, WV, *Intelligencer* and the Political Graveyard database. In addition, Mr. Forbes provided the names of those pharmacy students who were killed in action in World War II, whose deaths were unknown to me. Nancy Stewart at the Beckley, WV, *Register-Herald* and Carey Loch of Rutgers University graciously provided difficult to find newspaper articles. My thanks to Pam Johnson and Vicky Terry of the McClintic Public Library in Marlinton, WV, for their time searching for newspaper articles about Senator Allen. I am indebted to Jane Price Sharp, former editor of the *Pocahontas Times,* for her personal comments about Senator Fred Allen and for providing his obituary and biography from the 1955 *West Virginia Blue Book.*

After action reports of the 358 Infantry Regiment, 90th Infantry Division, were provided by staff at the National Archives, College Park, Maryland. I truly appreciate the assistance of Betsy Halki who provided Dr. Dennis Barber's eulogy of her late husband General Jack Halki; Colonel Don Patton and Vicki Rockis, who provided documents regarding Lieutenant Edward Rockis; and Dr. Mason R. Schaefer, military historian at the U.S. Army Center of Military History, who provided the unpublished manuscript, "Military Impact of the German V-Weapons" that contributed to the account of Major Rafferty's death. Additionally, I am deeply grateful to the following veterans for sharing their memories and their insight: Ralph Stevenson, Clyde Eugene Reed, James W. Fredlock, Ben Mitchell, and Leo Knowlton. I am indebted to the late Jean Plummer, Charles Rangos, Paula Corley (archives technician, National Personnel Records Center, St. Louis, MO), and Lt. Col. Thomas M. Jones (U.S. Army Human Resources Command,

Alexandria, VA). I thank Congressman Alan B. Mollohan and his staff for their thoughtful assistance.

Oral histories by Mayors Lydia Main, Richard Romig, Jr., Al Carolla, Tom Carson, Sam Kapourales, as well as Betty Jo Bare and Mary Turner (widows of Mayors Elwood Bare and Jim Turner) provided invaluable information about West Virginia municipal government in years gone by. I thank George Karos who provided the unpublished Natalie Martinez manuscript, "The Makings of a Mayor," on file at Shepherd University at Shepherdstown, WV; Bridgeport City Clerk Judy Lawson and City Treasurer Keith Boggs who made material contributions regarding Mayor Carl Furbee, Jr.'s administration of Bridgeport; and Paul Turman, Sr. and Dick Jefferson who addressed Huntington Mayor Plyburn's administration. Douglas Hilton and Virginia Yates' privately published book, *History of Ronceverte*, provided interesting supplemental information about the administration of Ronceverte Mayor Elwood Bare. I appreciate learning the unique story of George Rice's pharmacy registration from B. J. Payne, Assistant Executive Director of the WV Board of Pharmacy, and thank Gladys Bart Wandell and Debra Herndon (Shinnston City Clerk) for their contributions to the George Rice story. J.J. Finlayson's book, *Shinnston Tornado*, is a remarkable secondary source for this disaster. Lastly, I thank John Veasey of the Fairmont *Times West Virginian* for providing the file photograph of Jim Turner.

My warmest thanks to Senator Herbert Traubert's children: Joan Traubert Hooper, his daughter, who kindly provided the Blanche McDowell Neff columns from the Wellsburg, WV, *Daily Herald,* the John Kirker column from the *Wheeling Intelligencer*, and Senator Kilgore's telegram to Sen. Traubert; and Dick Traubert, his son, for his detailed discussion of the 1960 Presidential Campaign of Senator John F. Kennedy.

I appreciate Sally Stein of the National Association of Boards of Pharmacy for providing documents related to my late colleague, John P. Plummer. My warmest thanks to the late Stephen Crawford, who died unexpectantly in 2007, Thomas Menighan, now CEO of APhA, Joy Piper, senior administrative assistant (WVU School of Pharmacy), and Julie Murdock-Russo (University of Cincinnati Medical Center) for their assistance in preparing Chapter 9. The National Community Pharmacists Association kindly provided statistical data for Chapter 10. Paul Logsdon, director of alumni affairs at Ohio Northern University, graciously supplied archival data pertaining to Stephen Alfred Walker and the early years of the West Virginia State Pharmaceutical Association. I thank Willard Phillips for his help organizing the history of the "Dixon Affair." Carroll Martin, Ann Bond Smith, Jack Neale and Martha Hickman are appreciated for sharing their time in preparing Chapter 10, as did the late Jean Plummer. Cheryl Zeno of the Auditor's Office and Leigh of the Recorder's Office of Belmont County, OH, whose surname is unknown to me, are appreciated for their efforts spent researching records of E. Bruce Dawson. Joy Piper graciously provided the curricula vitae of Deans Louis A. Luzzi, S. Alan Rosenbluth and George R. Spratto.

Rosemary Raczko, manager of academic services of the University of Michigan College of Pharmacy, is greatly appreciated for reviewing records of J. Lester Hayman. I enjoyed great support from the current WVU pharmacy faculty Calvin Brister, Marie Abate, Arthur Jacknowitz and Dean Patricia Chase, as well as former Deans Sidney A. Rosenbluth and George R. Spratto. Former professors John W. Mauger, now dean at the University of Utah College of Pharmacy, and John H. Baldwin, currently associate dean at Nova Southeastern University College of Pharmacy, were gracious with their time. I thank former Dean Robert D'Alessandri of the WVU School of Medicine for providing the School of Medicine Annual Reports and Reports of the Liaison Committee on Medical Education for 1988.

My warmest thanks to Clarke Ridgway, Robert R. Lewis, Ann Bond Smith, Tom Traubert, and emeritus faculty Frank O'Connell, David Riley, James K. Lim, Carl Malanga and Louise Wojcik, the wife of Albert Wojcik, for their help in preparing the chapter on emeritus faculty. Lou Marcy, alumni coordinator at The Ohio State University College of Pharmacy, was a great source of information. Likewise, Ernest W. Turner, Charles V. Selby, Jr., Carol Ann Hudachek, Donley W. Hutson, the late Steve Crawford, Tom Carson, Lora Ann Good, Anita Henry of the Reference Department of the Raleigh (WV) Public Library, Senator Charles C. Lanham, Frances Fruth, Thomas Menighan and Sandra Justice generously assisted me in researching Chapter 10.

The chapter, Women as Leaders in the Profession, was greatly facilitated by three current School of Pharmacy faculty: Marie Abate, "Ginger" Scott, and Elizabeth Scharman; by seven community pharmacists: Lydia Main, Barbara Smith, Patty Johnston, Sandra Justice, Karen Reed, Carol Hudachek, and Susan Meredith; and by Dan Rider who provided the story of Alice Bennett. Peggy King, Felice Joseph, Elizabeth Keyes, and Michele McNeill are truly appreciated for donating their time to this project as well as their service to West Virginia.

I recognize the efforts of Brenda and Buddy Quertinmont for arranging interviews with Willie Akers, Clark "Hot Rod" Hundley, and Jerry West, each of whom provided information pertaining to Ann Dinardi. Special thanks are also due to Charles D. Chico, Sylvester Dinardi, Mary Angotti, Thomas David Gerkin, Mary Louise Gerkin, Clarke Ridgway, and former basketball Coach Gale Catlett for sharing their insights about Ann Dinardi with me.

I received inestimable help in researching the facts for the southern West Virginia floods of 2001 and 2002 from Eva (Stump) Burns, Ethel Lusk, Al Carolla, Arvel Wyatt, Jim Burks, Steve Crawford, and Steve Judy. Milton Proudfoot and Ruby Baumgartner provided valuable information about the 1985 Rowlesburg flood. John L. Finlayson's book, *Shinnston Tornado,* was a secondary source for the storm damage at Shinnston. I owe an immense debt to those pharmacists who assisted me in developing the story of the changing roles of pharmacists in Chapter 13: pharmacist-physicians Michael Cunningham, Judie Charlton, Bob Beto and Jimmy Mangus; pharmacist-attorneys Brian Gallagher, Stephen Brooks, Karen Kahle and Andrea Miller; and pharmacist-scientists Anna Maria Calcagno, Paula Stout and Alice Pau. Dean Dominick Purpura of the Albert Einstein College of Medicine was particularly gracious with his assistance in developing the story of Frank Lilly, as was Dr. Abraham I. Habenstreit, director of the Philip and Rita Rosen Department of Communications and Public Affairs of Yeshiva University. My thanks to James Coleman and the Reverend John Cooper-Martin for their help with research on pharmacists who become ministers. Additionally, I express my appreciation to Valerie Schmidt Mondelli, Jan Burks Skelton, Thomas Menighan and Michele McNeill for sharing their time and expertise for the section on entrepreneurs. Brenda Higa's (Program Assistant WVU School of Pharmacy) expertise in providing artwork, tables, and figures is noted and particularly appreciated. I thank Richard Stevens, executive director of the West Virginia Pharmacists Association and his administrative assistant, Susan Jones, for their kind assistance along the way. Susan has been a tremendous resource throughout this endeavor, never failing to take the time to assist me with my research. I appreciate the cooperation of each individual who was interviewed. If anyone has not been recognized the omission is mine alone, and I offer my apologies.

I wish to thank West Virginia University history graduate student Bryan Coyle for creating the Notes section, and Professor Eve Faulkes and her enthusiastic students (in particular Andrew Bernard) from the WVU College of Creative Arts for designing the cover art. Brian Jimmie and Gina Slaugenhoup of the WVU School of Medicine Alumni Office are greatly appreciated for their help on multiple occasions, in particular for their assistance in locating and editing photographs. Professor Pat Connor's advice related to chapter organization is likewise appreciated. Jeff McCorsky, assistant city manager of the City of Mogantown, merits acknowledgement for providing former Mayor Charles Blissitt's photograph. The assistance of Charles Woolcock, former finance director of the City of Morgantown is also noted. I wish to thank my son William H. Glover, Ellen Gambrill, and Dr. Dennis Worthen for kindly reading and providing a critique of this manuscript. I truly appreciate Dr. Worthen's preface. Finally, I want to recognize five wonderful people without whom this work could not have come to fruition: Dean George Spratto who initially suggested the project and provided encouragement along the way, my secretary Debbie Anderson, Amy Newton was invaluable in getting the manuscript into press, and Professors Marie Abate and Arthur Jacknowitz for their extraordinary patience and perseverance as editors, advisors, critics and friends.

Part One

Coming of Age

Chapter One

Through the Eyes
of Yesterday

Pharmacy in West Virginia has gradually changed over the past two centuries, moving from a product oriented to a service oriented profession. Contributing to this change was the evolution of drug manufacturing and distribution, expanded pharmacist education, emergence of professional organizations, and the growth of governmental influence. Specialty and subspecialty pharmacy practices have vastly increased the professional opportunities for today's pharmacist that did not exist in the past, and pharmacy practice has changed accordingly. This chapter briefly reviews these and other influences that have affected West Virginia pharmacy practice through the years.

The 18th and 19th Centuries

Present day West Virginia pharmacy practice has come a long way since its inauspicious beginnings in colonial days. In his 1946 treatise, *The Annals of Pharmacy in West Virginia*, Dr. Roy Bird Cook traced West Virginia pharmacy from its origins to World War II. In the 18th century, most of present-day West Virginia was located in a single county in Virginia, Augusta County. Four of Augusta County's earliest settlers who embodied the spirit of things to come were "physician-apothecaries:" Dr. William Fleming, who served as a military surgeon-apothecary during the battle of Point Pleasant (VA) in 1774; Dr. Adam Stephen, founder of the city of Martinsburg which was chartered in 1778; Dr. William McMechin, a naval medical officer who served on the first steamboat to navigate the Potomac River at Shepherdstown in December 1787; and Dr. Jessee Bennett, who in 1796 settled in Point Pleasant from the valley of Virginia, where he had performed the first Caesarean section in the United States two years earlier.[1]

By 1800, the population of Augusta County had grown enough to be divided into 13 counties. Shepherdstown was the location of western

Virginia's first drug store operated by physician-apothecary Robert Fahrrey. Dr. Fahrrey's store was soon followed by Dr. Charles Harper's store, advertised as an apothecary in the *Martinsburg (VA) Gazette* in December 1813. The concept of a store was a significant departure from the 19th century practice of dispensing drugs from saddlebags by horse-riding physician-apothecaries. Commonly prescribed treatments then in use were sulphur and lard to treat "the itch," compounds containing the oil of a polecat, bear, or snake for arthritic pain, phlebotomy (bleeding) for the treatment of pleurisy, and charms made from the blood of a black cat to treat headache, tooth ache, or erysipelas. Dr. Cook tells us that, "scarcely [was] a black cat to be seen whose ears and tail had not been cropped for a contribution of blood."

By 1839, Wheeling, Virginia — then known as the "Gateway to the West" — had grown to a population of nearly 9,000 and was home to nine druggists and chemists. With the arrival of the Baltimore and Ohio Railroad in 1852 Wheeling became a transportation hub to the west, and the *Wheeling (then Virginia) Intelligencer,* western Virginia's first newspaper, provided news from the east. By 1853, the number of pharmacies in western Virginia was rapidly increasing. In addition to those in Wheeling, Martinsburg, Charles Town and Harpers Ferry each had three pharmacies, Shepherdstown had two, and Charleston and Weston had one each. With the start of the Civil War, the Confederate states passed laws exempting druggists from military service, causing hundreds of imposters to claim membership in the profession to avoid serving in the war. Since western Virginia was largely in Union territory, however, this was not a problem in the future West Virginia. Drug stores provided service to belligerents on both sides in the Civil War depending on which army was in command of the area at the time.[1]

The late 1800s produced several "firsts" for pharmacy in what was now West Virginia. In 1872, Edwin L. Boggs of Charleston was the first West Virginian to attend a national pharmacy meeting, 21 years after the American Pharmaceutical Association was founded. As a result of interest shown by a number of Wheeling druggists, a bill to form a board of pharmacy passed the West Virginia legislature on February 21, 1881. Future board members were designated "Commissioners of Pharmacy," with "one man per congressional district [appointed who had] five years of drug store experience." But the wording of this legislation was somewhat vague and open to interpretation. Some assumed incorrectly that the stated membership requirement of "one man" meant only males were eligible for commission membership.

However, the bill specifically stated that fees collected by the Commissioners of Pharmacy were to fund an as yet unformed state pharmaceutical association, open for membership to all pharmacists in the state.

On June 1, 1881, about a hundred druggists from around the state met in Wheeling to organize the new pharmacy association and adopt a constitution. A Committee of Arrangements was named, chaired by Edmund Bocking. Its purpose was to arrange for a first convention in West Virginia. A constitution was adopted that declared the intent of the meeting was "to unite the reputable pharmacists and druggists of this state for mutual assistance and improvement." Samuel Laughlin, a wholesale druggist of the steel manufacturing family, was elected president. After electing officers, then Governor Jacob Jackson addressed the convention and heralded a "new day" for West Virginia pharmacy. During its early years the association met concurrently with the Commissioners at different West Virginia cities. However, in 1885 due to an apparent decline in interest by its members, the association disbanded. The Board of Commissioners was renamed the Board of Pharmacy and from 1885 to 1906 was the only active pharmacy organization in West Virginia.[1]

In 1901, the Board met at Parkersburg, where 20 candidates were examined. The minutes of the meeting recorded that "a number of the druggists praying for the exchange of certificates of the West Virginia and Ohio Boards was presented" but after some discussion the Board considered this inadvisable. Perhaps the Board members in attendance little appreciated the historic significance of their actions, but reciprocity with other states was first considered at this meeting, leading to the birth of the National Association of Boards of Pharmacy, which among its numerous responsibilities serves as an instrument for reciprocity.

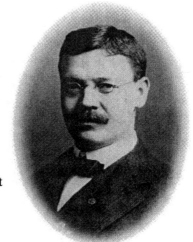

The 20ᵗʰ Century

Reorganization of the West Virginia Pharmaceutical Association

Dr. James Hartley Beal, who resided west of the Ohio River and was a former president of the American Pharmaceutical Association, observed the decline of interest in a state association by West Virginia pharmacists.

Dr. James Hartley Beal

As Dean of Scio College of Pharmacy (in Scioto County, Ohio, about 200 miles from Wheeling), he was interested in West Virginia pharmacy since many of his students were native West Virginians. Dr. Beal sent a letter to 30 of West Virginia's leading pharmacists announcing a meeting to be held in Parkersburg in October 1906. At that meeting, Dr. Beal addressed the attendees and stressed the need for a pharmacy organization and described the work of a state association. The proceedings were mailed to every known pharmacist in the state, resulting in the formation of a rejuvenated West Virginia Pharmaceutical Association.

The first annual convention of the new Association was held in Wheeling in June 1907. Dr. Beal selected speakers who were luminaries in the profession, including delegates to the National Association of Retail Druggists (NARD), faculty from the School of Pharmacy in Pittsburgh, and Mr. William E. Weiss, an entrepreneur from Wheeling (see Chapter 2). At the convention, Dr. Beal discussed a bill written earlier that month and signed into law by the governor. With flamboyant rhetoric, Dr. Beal informed the audience, "After waiting until many years behind the times in pharmaceutical legislation, this state has at a single bound placed itself among the states having modern and comprehensive laws for the regulation of pharmacy." West Virginia's new law required that prescriptions be filled only by pharmacists, addressed the improper sale of narcotics, and specified the governor would appoint Board of Pharmacy members.

One hundred forty-two new members were elected to membership at the 1907 Association convention. Of that number, Willa Hood Strickler was the only female applicant.[1] When Willa announced she wanted to join the Association, the secretary said, "You mean your husband wants to join — women are not eligible to join this organization!" Such was the greeting Willa received. Nonetheless, West Virginia's first woman pharmacist prevailed and was accepted, albeit grudgingly, as a member of the fledgling organization.

In June 1915, the ninth annual convention of the West Virginia Pharmaceutical Association was held in Clarksburg. Dr. J. N. Simpson, then president of West Virginia University, was the featured speaker. His topic, "The Mutual Dependence of the Druggist and Physician," is of interest today since it called for greater inter-professional teamwork to improve patient care.[1] Professor Charles H. Rogers (Ph.D. in pharmacy from the School of Medicine at WVU) followed with a discussion about the new Department of Pharmacy being formed at West Virginia University, a predecessor of the College of Pharmacy (now the School of Pharmacy) at WVU.

Interest in the West Virginia Pharmaceutical Association (WVPA) steadily increased following its reorganization. In 1916, the convention was held at Deer Park, Maryland, a popular resort location of that era, and it was the first of five annual meetings to be held beyond the West Virginia border. However, an international event was about to lead to another near collapse of the organization. The United States entered World War I in 1917, and by the following year, nearly every pharmacy in the state had been directly or indirectly affected by the war. Most pharmacy employees, pharmacists as well as clerks, were male, young, and subject to military service. The O. J. Stout pharmacy in Parkersburg, probably the most severely affected, lost 21 employees to the armed services. Pharmacy education at West Virginia University was likewise affected: Assistant Professor Rogers left his position at WVU for the University of Minnesota (where he developed a reputation of national prominence) and Instructor Bergy, the sole remaining faculty member in the Department, was called to active duty in the Army Chemical Corps. Bergy's departure caused the Department of Pharmacy to close for the duration of the war. When the state Association

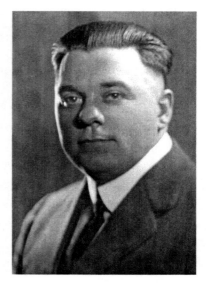

Gordon A. Bergy, circa 1919

next convened in June 1918, a mere 25 members attended and the speaker (an attorney from NARD) discussed war taxes and regulations imposed on pharmacists by the conflict. Although the war ended in November 1918, the taxes endured and talk about them dominated the state conventions until the tax on soft drinks was finally repealed in 1924.[1]

Merchandising and salesmanship became the dominant themes of WVPA conventions for the next two decades. In the "Roaring Twenties," money and ways to make money became the national rage. Edmund McGarry, a professor of business and economics at WVU, spoke at the 1924 convention on "Teaching the Management of Retail Stores," and the following year an address was given on "How to Increase Your Average Sale." Pharmaceutical manufacturers entered the arena by providing motivational speakers on sales enhancement to the Association in the latter 1920s. Examples of their speeches include: "Making More Money out of Retailing" in 1926 by a speaker provided by the Eli Lilly Company and "Modern Merchandizing in Drug Stores" in 1930 provided by the Parke-Davis Company. As the nation entered the "Great Depression," Mr. J. Gibbons Keech of Philadelphia discussed "Candy as an Income Builder for the Druggist." In 1933, when the depression showed no sign of moderating, the featured speaker's topic asked a prescient question, "Is the Independent Druggist Doomed?"

Pharmacists were not commissioned in the armed services during World War I, although many became sergeants or pharmacist mates in charge of medical dispensaries. They helped compensate for the shortage of medical officers at that time without receiving either the appropriate rank or pay. During the peacetime years from 1919 to 1941, the plight of the military pharmacist was either neglected or ignored. The profession in 1942, as it had been in 1917, was unprepared to take up the fight for a professional role for its pharmacist members. A Pharmacy Corps and a Medical Administrative Corps (MAC) had been organized in 1920 but largely functioned in the areas of supply and administration. Service-trained technicians, products of a brief 'count and pour' course, filled prescriptions. Essentially, pharmacists lacked a professional role in the United States Army during the Second World War. In both 1943 and 1944, the WVPA convention was reduced to a single day conference, during which the programs consisted solely of a discussion of the pharmacist's plight in the armed forces. Due to wartime restrictions such as gasoline rationing, no convention was held in 1945.

Following the Japanese attack on Pearl Harbor in December 1941, West Virginia pharmacists faced problems similar to those encountered in 1917-1918. As younger males once again entered the armed services, help for the older pharmacy-owner became difficult to find. Overnight, clerks and soda fountain employees shifted gender, from male to female, reversing a trend of male dominance antedating to the early nineteenth century. Convention programs again addressed war issues rather than merchandizing and sales. For the duration of the war the pharmacist was a major contributor to the war effort, serving in ways never dreamed of during peacetime.

Pharmacies became centers for tin collection, with showcase displays publicizing the need for the metal in war production. Customers were taught that each submarine needed more than three tons of tin, a heavy bomber required 48 pounds of tin, and each medium tank, 35 pounds.[2] Customers turned in their empty toothpaste and shaving cream tubes at pharmacies, and pharmacists encouraged their patients to invest the change from their purchases in war stamps that were convertible into war bonds. Many pharmacists donned the hat of air raid wardens or otherwise participated in civilian defense activities. Overnight, quinine disappeared from prescription shelves as pharmacists contributed to the National Quinine Pool to combat malaria in the armed forces.

The Era of Count and Pour

Following the discovery of penicillin in the late 1930s, other antibiotics and entirely new classes of therapeutic agents such as psychotherapeutic drugs, corticosteroids, cardioactive medications, antihypertensive agents, and oral contraceptives came into being. Unlike pharmacy of the past that had focused on symptomatic relief of minor illnesses, during the first three decades following World War II pharmacy became a bastion of prevention and cure for serious diseases. Soda fountains became relics of the past. Chain stores and groceries, eager to compete for the prescription dollar, became a threat to the independent pharmacy. With the advent of new single entity therapies, compounded prescription use fell precipitously. In the 1930s, the majority of prescriptions were compounded. In 1960, one in 25 prescriptions was compounded. By 1970, only one in 100 required compounding.[3] The pharmaceutical industry invested vast sums of money on research and development of new drug entities. As the potency of new drugs escalated, so did their potential to cause harm. Drastic changes followed in pharmacy practice. As the potential for toxicity increased, so did governmental control. The Food, Drug, and Cosmetic act of 1938 required proof of safety of a therapeutic entity. The Durham-Humphrey amendment to the Food, Drug, and Cosmetic Act of 1952 followed, making a clear separation between prescription and nonprescription drugs. It specifically recognized the legitimacy of prescription refills, the legitimacy of telephoned prescriptions, and required the indication of a specific number of prescription refills. The Harris-Kefauver Drug amendments of 1962 required proof of efficacy and clearly delineated a methodology for clinical trials. Finally, the Omnibus Reconciliation Act of 1990 (OBRA 90) required patient counseling in entitlement programs such as Medicaid. OBRA 90 not only increased the pharmacist's responsibility to educate patients, it added both prospective and retrospective drug utilization review that further enhanced their professional role. It was both reasonable and imperative that pharmacy education be expanded accordingly.

The University of Southern California introduced the first Doctor of Pharmacy degree program in 1950. National change, however, was slow.

Most U.S. schools of pharmacy only moved to a five-year Bachelor of Science in pharmacy degree by 1960, followed by a shift to a Doctor of Pharmacy (Pharm.D.) program evolving gradually over the next four decades with emphasis on the role of the clinical or patient oriented pharmacist. At West Virginia University, an add-on Pharm.D. degree program was first provided in 1994 for those with a Bachelor of Science in pharmacy degree. The current entry-level Pharm.D. program was introduced in 1998. One of the most drastic changes occurring with the era of clinical pharmacy expansion involved the role of the hospital pharmacist. No longer relegated to the basement, the hospital pharmacy took on added responsibilities as decentralized pharmacists became integral members of the health care team. Decentralized pharmacists usually attend patient rounds with the medical staff as drug therapy experts and actively promote medication safety, resulting in dramatically improved patient care. While change has been slower coming in the community pharmacy setting, many examples of innovative, patient-centered retail pharmacy practices that offer disease state management programs and specialized compounding services exist in West Virginia.

The Gender Shift

Prior to World War II, pharmacy was considered a "man's profession." The hours of pharmacy operation were one reason for this gender disproportion. Community pharmacies of that era remained open from 8 AM until 10 PM with only a clerk and pharmacist on night duty. In addition to the 14 hour workday, concern about robbery or assault *en route* home were realistic and dissuaded women from becoming community pharmacists. By 1950, an artificial divide had developed, with women migrating to the hospital and men to the "corner drug store." However, studies of pharmacy economics failed to justify the customary hours of operation characterizing the community pharmacy. Also, the shift from ownership of independent pharmacies to employees of chain pharmacies resulted in less business involvement and greater flexibility of hours. As hours decreased, the gender disparity between hospital and community pharmacy began to fade. As shown in Figure 1, the number of women entering the pharmacy profession in West Virginia began an upward trend during World War II (when men were in the military service), plateaued from the 1940s to the 1970s, and then began to escalate. By the late 1980s, women dominated the profession with those graduating in the 1980s and 1990s accounting for over 50% of all female graduates from 1920 onward.

Learning From Our Past

Looking back at the winding road West Virginia pharmacy has traveled shows us that change is both inevitable and ongoing. Neither pharmacy nor medicine can advance patient care in a vacuum. As observed by WVU President Simpson in 1915, the sister professions of medicine and pharmacy are closely intertwined. Changes occur in concert, with each advance in medicine necessitating a similar change in pharmacy. As illustrated in Chapter 2, pharmacists advanced herbal medicine use by developing novel delivery systems and introducing innovative marketing techniques. Governmental bodies reacted by legislating new laws and regulations to protect the public at large. The pharmaceutical industry introduced research, resulting in the development of more efficacious drugs while limiting toxicity.

The era of professional competition is past. Pharmacists and physicians no longer compete for patients or the sale of drugs. As the momentum of change continues to accelerate, the forces for competition will dissipate and complementary forces will prevail. Will West Virginia pharmacy be ready for the future? A look at our history tells us "yes."

Figure 1

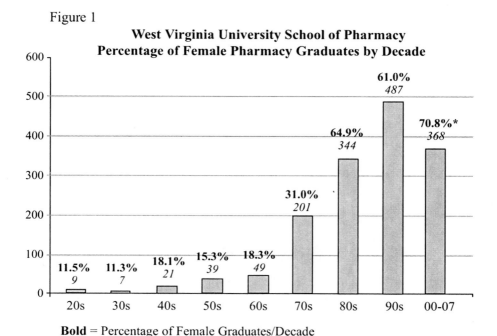

West Virginia University School of Pharmacy
Percentage of Female Pharmacy Graduates by Decade

Bold = Percentage of Female Graduates/Decade
Italics = Total Number of Female Graduates/Decade
* = Percentage based on graduates thus far this decade

Chapter Two

From a Small Town to the World Stage

Willliam Erhard Weiss started from humble beginnings. Born December 18, 1879 in Canton, Ohio, he was the son of German emigrants. He studied pharmacy at the Philadelphia College of Pharmacy and Science (now the Philadelphia College of Pharmacy) and graduated after two years of study in 1892 with a Ph.G. degree.[1] Following graduation, William settled in Sistersville, a small town in West Virginia along the Ohio River, where he worked at a local pharmacy, Hendershott's Drug Store. William, however, had loftier ambitions than to be a small town druggist. According to Henry O. Boette, a contemporary pharmacist from Huntington, WV, Weiss "had a wild idea about starting a drug firm" to manufacture and sell patent medicines.[2] He decided to put his plan into action with his childhood friend, Albert H. Diebold. Together they traveled around the northern panhandle of West Virginia on a horse-drawn buckboard hawking their first product, a headache remedy they called Neuralgine which presumably contained acetanilide, a chemical analgesic of that era.[3] Buoyed by their success in this venture, they formed and incorporated the *Neuralgyline Company* in Wheeling, WV, a town 45 miles north of Sistersville, to manufacture and market their product.[4]

Most patent medicine companies in the early 1900s marketed single products. No studies of efficacy or safety were required to market a product. If undertaken at all, the inventor self-administered it to test for safety. Sales of such nostrums normally declined as the public learned they were not effective. When that occurred, the manufacturer had three options: come up with a new product, close the business, or move to another venue. To circumvent this potential problem, Weiss and Diebold decided to form a conglomerate to manufacture products of a diverse nature. Should sales of one product decline, profits from other products would keep the company afloat. In support of this concept, they began to acquire small patent medicine companies to expand their product line.

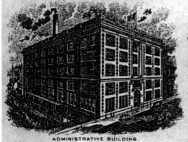
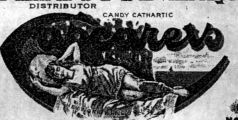
Cascarets Advertisement

12

One early acquisition was the *Knowlton Danderine Company*, purchased for its dandruff-remover product, Double Danderine. In 1902, Weiss and Diebold paid $22,000 for a controlling interest in the J. W. Janes Company, the manufacturer of several proprietary products including a headache powder. In 1909, Weiss and Diebold purchased the common stock as well as control of the Attica, Illinois based *Sterling Remedy Company*, manufacturer of Cascarets and NO-TO-BAC. Cascarets were candy-flavored laxatives, advertised for children's use (see advertisement) and touted to be harmless. NO-TO-BAC was a smoking cessation remedy that presumably contained lobeline, an herbal remedy known as Indian tobacco with effects similar to nicotine. Since NO-TO-BAC users tended toward constipation, Weiss and Diebold acquired the *California Fig Syrup Company* for its laxative product, Syrup of Figs. As noted by Plummer and Mann,[3] products manufactured by Weiss and Diebold tended to be synergistic, in that a side effect of one product could be alleviated by a second.[5]

Weiss was impressed with the word "sterling" and considered it of enormous importance as a corporate name. Within five years, the company was worth $500,000 and further increased to $4 million by 1912. After acquiring the *Sterling Remedy Company*, the name of the *Neuralgyline Company* was changed to *Sterling Products Company* and was incorporated in 1917. Weiss served as the CEO of the rapidly growing *Sterling Products, Inc.* conglomerate. Capital stock, initially valued at $1,000, appreciated rapidly. Weiss and Diebold thus demonstrated their acumen as astute businessmen as well as successful entrepreneurs.[3] From the beginning, their goal was to make money, and make money they did.

Meanwhile, across the Atlantic, events were unfolding that would profoundly impact Weiss' world. A young and aggressive German company, *Farbenfabriken Bayer*, was branching out from its well-established dye manufacturing business into the more lucrative area of pharmaceuticals. A by-product of dye manufacture was para-nitrophenol, a compound structurally similar to acetanilid. This waste product of no apparent utility was stored in barrels behind their manufacturing plant, creating a problem of disposal. However, their chemists discovered that para-nitrophenol could be converted to acetophenitidin, a chemical with analgesic properties. Bayer's scientists thus "conceived, developed, tested" and now prepared to market a pharmaceutical product they trademarked as Phenacetin, made exclusively from the waste material from the dye making process.[3] Bayer had ushered in the dawn of the modern pharmaceutical industry by linking dye manufacture to the production of drugs.

It is axiomatic that profit drives research and research drives industry. *Farbenfabriken Bayer* now owned both the patent and the trademark for Phenacetin in the U.S., Germany and Great Britain. Clinically, Phenacetin (acetophenitidin) appeared to be more effective than acetanilid, and although it was toxic, its toxicity was less. Thus, the new drug was considered an improvement over acetanilid. Since acetophenitidin was synthesized from industrial waste, it was inexpensive to produce requiring no raw materials to be purchased or developed. In addition, *Farbenfabriken Bayer* charged more for Phenacetin than its predecessor. As a result, their profit was huge. *Farbenfabriken Bayer's* innovative product had great potential for success.[4] Now all *Farbenfabriken Bayer* lacked was public demand for their product.

Aspirin was in common usage throughout the world, providing the potential for a worldwide market. *Farbenfabriken Bayer* manufactured aspirin, but because acetylsalicylic acid had first been synthesized in 1853, it was not entitled to a patent. However, a trademark could be registered.[5] By use of a distinctive trademark in conjunction with persuasive advertising, the public could be convinced that Bayer Aspirin was superior to other manufacturers' products. *Farbenfabriken Bayer's* motive in promoting Bayer Aspirin was more to advance its trade name, Bayer, as a household name than to sell aspirin.

However, war clouds were gathering over Europe and on April 6, 1917, after several years of neutrality, the United States entered World War I against Germany. Six months later Congress passed the "Trading with the Enemy Act," an act that when signed into law permitted the Office of Alien Property Custodian to take enemy property in the United States and hold it in trust until the end of the war. An amendment to the act authorized the U.S. government to seize enemy intellectual property (patents, copyrights and trademarks) as well. As a result, *Farbenfabriken Bayer* lost control of the Bayer trademark and their manufacturing facility in the United States.

Weiss had learned about Bayer and, after the war, Weiss/Sterling Products petitioned the Board of Trade to purchase the assets of the *Bayer Company, Ltd.* in Great Britain. The sale was approved and in May 1920, *Sterling Products Inc.* became owner of the Bayer patents and trademark in the United States, Canada, the British Commonwealth and certain Latin American countries. Sterling also acquired both the trademark and patent for Phenacetin in the U.S.

Negotiations for the terms of the purchase agreement in Germany, however, did not go as smoothly as they had in England and were contentious. Weiss made no friends among the German owners who felt he was "aggressive and brash." Several trips to Germany were required to hammer home an agreement, although eventually he prevailed. An employee at this time described Weiss as "…a guy from Wheeling, West Virginia" who was just "…a small town guy suddenly playing in the big leagues." [6]

After *Sterling Products* gained control of the Bayer trademark, the corporate headquarters was moved to New York City where Weiss occupied a suite on the top floor of an office building in Manhattan.[1] All ties to *Farbenfabriken Bayer* were severed. However, in 1928, the former German owners, in an attempt at reconciliation, presented Weiss with an honorary Doctor of Philosophiae degree from the University of Cologne. The ceremony was conducted entirely in German at the corporate headquarters in New York City.[7] Weiss, having never become proficient in German and unable to speak the language, made little effort to show his appreciation for the conciliatory effort. Nonetheless, to the end of his days he insisted on being addressed as "Doctor Weiss."

Unfortunately for Weiss, and rather ironically, his German ethnicity would become problematic. Between 1928 and the beginning of World War II, Weiss spent his time either traveling or in Wheeling. Although he maintained a winter residence in Florida and a summer home in Michigan, he did not like New York City and preferred the quiet lifestyle of West Virginia. As anti-German sentiment increased in the United States, the press began to denounce *Sterling Products* with messages that suggested, "Sterling was part of a [Nazi] program for the conquest of America." One such article ("These Firms

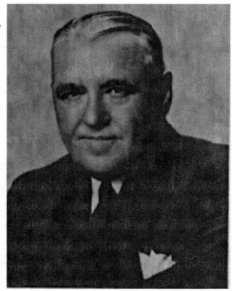

William E. Weiss

Earn Money") in the tabloid *PM* stated "Hitler gets millions for war chest through links with American firms. Sterling…would help Hitler win the Americas." Another story encouraged the U.S. President to freeze Sterling's funds, which would essentially shut down the company.[8]

The media frenzy was based on speculation rather than fact. Weiss had no formal ties to or expressed admiration for Germany. Weiss and *Sterling Products* were both involved in support of America's war effort during World War II. Weiss directed USO fund drives in Wheeling and served on the Chemical Warfare Board in Washington, D.C. during the war.[4] These activities went unrecognized.

As a result of the hue and cry of the media and negative public sentiment, the U.S. Justice Department became involved. Francis Biddle, a personal friend of President Franklin D. Roosevelt and the acting attorney general, began to investigate and the Treasury Department froze the firm's assets. Throughout the summer of 1941, the press and politicians fanned the fire. In September, both Mr. Weiss' brother and his daughter died. Weiss' world was falling apart; he feared a repeat of what happened in World War I when the federal government seized all intellectual property and corporate assets of foreign companies. One of his companies, Winthrop, was jointly owned by the U.S. branch of I. G. Farben, and, in theory, could be considered a German company. Francis Biddle's actions could cause him to lose all he had gained from a lifetime of work.

On September 3, 1941, under extreme duress, Mr. Weiss was forced to sign a consent decree. It stipulated that William E. Weiss and Albert Diebold were to be barred for life from *Sterling Products* and ordered to pay the government $5,000 and $1,000 in fines, respectively. By signing that decree Weiss had lost everything: his factories, his companies, and his fortune. Weiss retreated to his Wheeling office and he refused to vacate it until December. As the ultimate insult, when he left his office to take a vacation his belongings were tossed out into the parking lot. He later traveled through the midwest and spent time with his daughter's children who had moved in with him after their mother's death.

On Tuesday afternoon, September 1, 1942, Weiss' chauffeur driven automobile collided with another vehicle at Harbor Springs, Michigan. Dr. and Mrs. Weiss had been spending the summer at their home on Indian River at Columbus Beach, Michigan. He was thrown against the frame of the automobile, sustaining a fractured skull. He died the following afternoon without regaining consciousness. The cause of death was determined to be an intracranial hemorrhage.[9] Funeral services were held on September 5 with burial in Wheeling.[10]

William E. Weiss was a small-town rural pharmacist who had played a major role on the world stage of pharmaceutical manufacturing. He was a successful industrialist, an entrepreneur, and a civic-minded individual. Weiss' empire had included multiple factories that provided jobs for thousands of people. Without doubt, he was a pharmacist who had made a difference in West Virginia and the world.

The story of Diebold, Weiss' boyhood friend and founding business partner, is a fascinating tale of success in its own right. Albert Henry Diebold was born January 13, 1873, in Canton, Ohio, and like Weiss, was a son of German immigrants. His parents had arrived in the United States as young, married adults. Albert was the sixth child and the third of four sons, all born in Ohio. Birth records reveal his name as Henry Albert Diebold, although throughout life he was known as Albert H. Diebold.[11] Albeit acclaimed as a pharmacist, little is known of Albert's education. He may have learned pharmacy as an apprentice without any formal pharmacy education, which was commonplace in that era.[12] Interviews with three members of his extended family failed to confirm an association of Albert Diebold to the profession of pharmacy.[13] Although a matter of conjecture, it is likely Albert was working for his older brother, Charles, at Diebold Safe and Lock Company in Canton while Weiss was studying pharmacy in Philadelphia.[14] In 1900 at age 27, he joined his friend William Weiss selling *Neuralgine* from a horse-drawn buckboard around West Virginia's northern panhandle.

When *Sterling Products Company* was incorporated in 1917, Diebold served as president, a position he held until his retirement in 1941.[15] He continued as a director of the company until the year before his death in 1964. In the Weiss-Diebold partnership at *Sterling Products*, Albert Diebold was considered to be the "money man" for his uncanny ability to select products considered superb financial opportunities, whereas Weiss was the "operations man." In acquiring small companies, Diebold selected products that were easy to manufacture, inexpensive to produce, readily distinguishable from the competition, and freely marketable. Under their management, *Sterling Products, Inc.* became the nation's first patent medicine conglomerate.[16]

In 1909, Weiss and Diebold began to acquire promising patent medicine companies, laying the groundwork for the future *American Home Products Company* that they both cofounded. Like *Sterling Products, Inc.,* it distributed over-the-counter products, particularly those with analgesic properties. An early acquisition was the John F. Murray Advertising Agency established by John Murray from Monroe, Iowa, who was known for his advertising acumen. Mr. Murray had previously worked for the Wrigley

Chewing Gum Company in Chicago. Together the three men formed a well functioning business utilizing each man's expertise: Weiss for his entrepreneurial skills, Diebold for his ability to select money-making products, and Murray for his advertising experience.[17] Over time, Albert Diebold acquired 25 proprietary companies for the *American Home Products Company*. He relied upon licensing rather than in-house drug discovery and commercialization to obtain products. Emphasis was placed on a strong profit performance rather than research and development.[18]

Prior to working for the Wrigley Company, John F. Murray had been a carnival sideshow barker. Murray found some of the tent show techniques to be of benefit in advertising. Half of the company's net income was invested in newspaper advertising and sales began to escalate. In 1922, John Murray designed a pocket-sized brochure to be kept in the family medicine cabinet "for easy reference." This was actually a thinly disguised advertisement for their eight leading products. Patent medicines such as *Jad Salts* ("a cleanser of the liver and bowels"), *Dr. August Koenig's Hamburg Breast Tea* ("a breaker of colds"), and *St. Jacobs Oil* ("a liniment for muscular pains and aches due to exertion or exposure") were thus touted to the general public in the privacy of their bathrooms.[18]

The trio next hired Stanley P. Jadwin, a wholesale druggist who thoroughly understood drug distribution. Jadwin's job was to attend pharmacy conventions and advise his associates of promising new products. He recommended they buy the Wyeth Chemical Company, makers of *Wyeth's Sage and Sulphur Compound*, a hair dye. Once acquired, Jadwin was named president and the company office was established in Murray's advertising agency office located in the Whitehall Building in lower Manhattan. Impressed by the Whitehall name that to Diebold implied prestige, they formed the *Whitehall Pharmacal Company* to serve as a marketing arm for their burgeoning business.

However, the four-man team needed someone to manufacture its products. Such a man was found in Detroit, Michigan. William H. Kirn was a highly respected pharmaceutical chemist who was head of the Formula Department of the Parke-Davis Company. Arrangements were made for their products to be manufactured at the Parke-Davis plant in Detroit under Kirn's supervision.[18]

Kirn recruited the sixth founder of the *American Home Products Company*, Walter B. Rowles. Rowles was an English-trained pharmaceutical chemist with an inventive mind who worked with Kirn at Parke-Davis. His area of expertise was the development of new products, of which the first was *Rowles Red Pepper Rub*, a counter-irritant ointment they advertised as a treatment for "arthritic pain, lumbago, neuritis, sciatica, backache, strains, colds and congestion."[18] With the six-man team in place, the time was right to initiate a national advertising campaign.

By 1925, *American Home Products Company* had marketed 25 proprietary products with total annual sales of greater than $1 million. Diebold and Weiss decided to consolidate their patent medicine companies under the roof of a single corporate entity. Anticipating ready acceptance of their proposed corporate structure by Wall Street investment bankers, they were dismayed when their proposal was rejected. The brokers and investment bankers considered the return on their annual sales insufficient for such a substantial initial public offering. To them, patent medicines and their companies were a risky business.[18]

In response, Albert Diebold began to search for a product that would ease the concerns of Wall Street. He learned the maker of *Petrolagar* was offering its ethical drug company (a manufacturer of prescription drugs) for sale. *Petrolagar* (mineral oil and agar gel used to treat stomach problems) was a moneymaker and its acquisition would greatly enhance the value of their company. His offer of $2,500,000 was accepted and the financiers agreed to the deal. Thus, *American Home Products Company* was incorporated February 4, 1926, with a corporate valuation of $2,900,000.

When Wall Street bankers rejected Diebold's corporate consolidation plan, he, Murray, and Kirn conducted a survey of pharmacists regarding their perception of the products produced by the *American Home Products Company*. The results of this survey indicated that pharmacists looked favorably on only four of their products.[18] To correct this problem, Mr. Murray designed displays for a number of their products and the poorest performers were discontinued. With a nationwide advertising campaign that resulted in an 80% rise in sales, *American Home Products'* stock rose from $30 per share in 1926 to $71 per share by the end of 1927.

Anacin, an analgesic product then containing acetylsalicylic acid, caffeine, and quinine sulfate, was purchased in 1930 from Van Ess Laboratories for two million dollars. This proprietary product was heavily promoted on radio. Interestingly, by the mid 1930s, Diebold found he was competing with himself. Anacin had become *American Home's* leading product, yet still trailed *Sterling Drug's* Bayer Aspirin in sales. As part of its advertising crusade, Anacin sponsored two-noontime serial programs broadcast on the CBS Radio Network Monday through Friday, "Romance of Helen Trent," followed by "Our Gal Sunday." These programs carried a message, directed to the American housewife, that three ingredients are better than one. "Anacin is compounded on the prescription principle, meaning it is a combination of medically proven and tested ingredients, not just one," the announcer would intone. Additionally, *American Home Products* spent another $200,000 a year to bring "Easy Aces," a family oriented radio situation comedy, to American families with a similar advertising message three nights a week.

Albert H. Diebold learned another lesson that he turned into profit when the investment bankers rejected his plan in 1925. Both he and Weiss had avoided owning ethical pharmaceutical companies because such companies were not adaptable to Diebold's four basic principles of easy to manufacture, inexpensive to produce, readily distinguishable from competitor's products, and freely marketable. Although each had amassed a fortune selling proprietary drugs, the fact that investment bankers considered these products risky was of concern. Thus, when Harvard University decided to liquidate their holdings in John Wyeth and Brother, an ethical pharmaceutical manufacturer without ties to the Wyeth Chemical Company they already owned, Diebold made an offer. The asking price was four million dollars, but the condition of the business was poor and Harvard was eager to sell. His offer of $2.9 million was promptly accepted.

By 1933, at the height of the depression, *American Home Products* was suffering financially. The company was top heavy with managers and the organizational structure was weak. Bookkeeping and accounting procedures were not being assiduously followed and the company president was in poor health. To address these problems, the Board of Directors appointed an Executive Committee to be chaired by Albert Diebold. The president voluntarily retired for health reasons, and Vice President Stanley Jadwin resigned as did the newly appointed president, Theodore E. Caruso.

Albert Diebold took a bold step and brought a Certified Public Accountant from *Sterling Drug Company* to take over the company. Alvin G. Brush was a different type of leader. He was familiar with *American Home Products,* having previously headed an accounting firm that handled their accounts as well as those from competing firms. Diebold was impressed with his analytical mind and when Brush was presented to the Board of Directors in April 1935, he was unanimously approved.[18] Henceforth, each product was evaluated and those that did not measure up by their value to the public or profitability were eliminated. Brush made an executive decision to replace a minimum of five percent of the products annually. Additionally, he assiduously avoided luxury items.

A sales force of pharmaceutical representatives was hired and trained to promote *American Home Products'* prescription products to physicians. Wyeth was changing its direction, moving from proprietary to prescription drugs. The company entered the field of vaccine development, the "cutting edge" of medicine at the time. By the end of the 1930s, *American Home Products* acquired a strong position in household product sales. EFF Laboratories was purchased for its vitamin business and the SMA baby food line was acquired. Specialty groceries provided a foothold in the food business and household products gave entry to hardware, department stores, and grocery chains.

American Home Products was a major force among pharmaceutical companies during World War II. With the invasion of Guadalcanal, the need for blood plasma, sulfonamides, quinine and Atabrine tablets for malaria, as well as dyes used in smoke grenades escalated. Wyeth employees received one of the first Army-Navy "E" Awards for manufacturing excellence. In all, Wyeth employees received four "E" Awards during World War II, equal to the number received by employees of the Winthrop Stearns Division of Sterling Drug. One of Wyeth's greatest contributions to the war effort was the mass production of penicillin. Wyeth made its initial shipment of penicillin to the armed forces in June 1943, one of the first drug companies to mass-produce this important antibiotic. In conjunction with Pfizer, Merck, Squibb, and other pharmaceutical manufacturers, the combined output of this antibiotic reached historic heights by 1945.

In his later years, Albert Diebold lived in Locust Valley, Long Island, NY, and maintained a winter home in Florida. He remained active in the Proprietary Association, a patent medicine trade group, and the Protestant Episcopal Church. An avid tennis enthusiast, he had memberships in several country and tennis clubs in both states. He gained renown as a discriminating collector of paintings and fine arts.[18] Albert H. Diebold retired in 1941, having assured himself the company was in good hands with Brush. He remained on the *American Home Products* Board of Directors until 1963, albeit ever vigilant. He died at age 91 on February 17, 1964, at his home in Florida.[16] With his death the Weiss-Diebold story, a tale of two boyhood friends in a small town with a simple idea they turned it into fortune and success, ended.

Part Two
Public Service

Chapter Three
Community Leaders and Mayors

Most citizens who desire to be mayor are civic-minded individuals motivated by a sense of community spirit, reinforced by a commitment to enhance the common good. In such a setting, the community pharmacist is a "natural" candidate for mayor and meets the specifications as well as or better than many other professionals. The community pharmacist is well-educated, knowledgeable in matters of community health, knows the citizens well and understands their problems and concerns. Unfortunately, the literature is devoid of data on pharmacist-mayors, with an exception of a brief communication published two decades ago.[1]

West Virginia is a small state with a low population density. According to 2000 census data, the largest city, Charleston, has a population of slightly more than 50,000, with a total population in the surrounding areas of 306,000.[2] As a result, professional politicians at the local level are relatively few. Seventeen West Virginia pharmacists have been elected mayor from 1921 to 2007, and they have won 63 elections. In fact, only three pharmacists have been defeated in their quest to become mayor in the past 86 years. Four individuals won 31 of the elections, each term encompassing two years, and the only woman among them has been reelected mayor 16 times.* Three of these four individuals have also been the only candidates to lose an election. Paradoxically, Mayor Lydia Main won her first election as a write-in candidate and the only contest she lost was to a write-in candidate.

The smallest cities in West Virginia have most commonly elected pharmacists as mayors. Nine of the 17 pharmacist-mayoral candidates were elected in cities with a population of 2,000 to 10,000; three candidates were elected in cities with a population between 10,000 and 50,000. Only four pharmacists have been elected mayor of municipalities classified as

---

A more detailed description of their accomplishments is found in Appendix A

towns or villages (population less than 2000), probably due to the paucity of pharmacists residing in these areas. One of these small-town mayors, however, won 16 contests resulting in three decades of public service.

There are more similarities than differences among the West Virginia pharmacist-mayors. Fifteen of the 17 pharmacist-mayors were independent

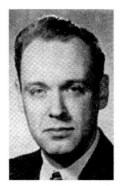

Donald Sinclair

pharmacy owners, nine were members of the Masonic lodge, and three were members of other fraternal organizations. Fourteen actively participated in community service organizations, of which 12 held leadership positions in either the Kiwanis, Rotary, Lions International, or the Chamber of Commerce. When Donald Sinclair, a mayor of Bethlehem, West Virginia died, his obituary was published on the front page of *The Wheeling Intelligencer*. Only one of its 33 paragraphs was devoted to his pharmacy practice, with the balance describing his public service and contributions as mayor.[3] In addition to leadership through governance, these pharmacist-mayors also demonstrated their leadership skills in business and professional organizations, with four having served the West Virginia Pharmacists Association (WVPA) as president.

George Karos, the current mayor of Martinsburg, is a prototypical West Virginia pharmacist-mayor. Over the years he has been recognized as a civic leader who served in a leadership position in several local and regional organizations. As a child, the future mayor grew up in a residence where Greek was the language of the home. In high school his friends called him "Squeaky Greek" because his sneakers squeaked when he dribbled the basketball down the court.[4]

Fred Allen first demonstrated his leadership skills as mayor of Marlinton from 1928 to 1932. Thereafter, he served the citizens of Pocahontas County's Twelfth District in the West Virginia State Senate (see Chapter 4). Senator Allen was appointed president pro tempore for the 1945, 1949, 1951, 1953, and 1955 sessions.[5, 6]

Benjamin H. Carson received an ROTC commission as second lieutenant upon graduation from pharmacy school in 1954. After completing his service obligation as an infantry officer, he and his brother Tom opened College Drug Store in 1956 where they practiced pharmacy together in Montgomery, West Virginia. Thirty-eight years later, after Ben's death, Tom sold the pharmacy and retired. In 1992, during his tenure as mayor of Montgomery, Ben was instrumental in obtaining the location for the Mount Olive Correctional Complex state penitentiary near Montgomery in Fayette County.

William Sidney Coleman joined the WVPA the year before he graduated from the Medical College of Virginia, part of Virginia Commonwealth University, School of Pharmacy in 1925. Bill Coleman served 22 years in Lewisburg city government, including six terms as mayor.

Carl E. Furbee, Jr., was a pharmacy leader with an extraordinary focus on goals and anticipated accomplishments. His energy was expended to support the three pillars of his professional career: his pharmacy practice, state association, and community. Carl Furbee served as president of the WVPA in 1965 – 1966 (see Chapter 10). His successes regarding the first two goals were rewarded in 1967 when he received the Outstanding Alumnus Award of the West Virginia University College of Pharmacy. His successes regarding the third goal are presented in Appendix A.

Samuel G. Kapourales is a former mayor of Williamson who continues to serve his state in various capacities. He was honored by the West Virginia State Medical Association in 1985 when he received the Medical Association's Presidential Citation for Outstanding Community Service as mayor and civic leader in Mingo County, West Virginia. No other pharmacist has received such recognition from the West Virginia State Medical Association.

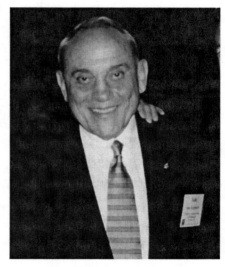

Lydia Main has been involved in politics much of her adult life. In addition to her three decades of service as Masontown's mayor, Lydia has served on numerous local, state, and national professional and civic organizations.[7] Lydia has defied the

Sam Kapourales

odds: she has practiced for 50 years in a community with a population of between 800 and 1000. Few communities with a population so small have a pharmacy. In fact, an individual recently died who had been her patient for a half century.

A mother of four daughters, Lydia reared each in the pharmacy. Through the years one of Lydia's on-going struggles was to keep her toddlers out of harms way. Her youngest daughter couldn't resist opening the boxes of band-aids. The second daughter zeroed in on the boxes of D-Con, but Lydia had trained the oldest child to take responsibility for protecting her younger sister from eating the rat poison. The third daughter liked to play clerk, and would pull items from the shelves to make a sale to the customer. As the years passed, one of Lydia's daughters died, and in doing so she left Lydia

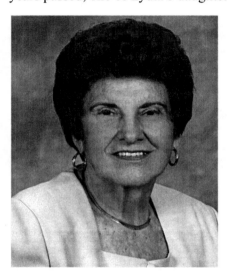

Lydia Main

with two granddaughters to rear. In all, Lydia reared six girls in the pharmacy, without doubt a first for West Virginia.

As mayor of Masontown, Lydia also has the responsibility of being "police judge," where she must mete out justice for miscreants such as speeders or drunks. Naturally, this transpires in the pharmacy; Main Pharmacy is the only pharmacy in the state (and possibly the nation) where police court is held in a community drug store. Lydia takes pride in her role of small town mayor. During her tenure as mayor, Masontown has acquired new water and sewage systems. She has served her citizens well.

William J. Plyburn owned his pharmacy in Barboursville, West Virginia, for almost 30 years. Like Lydia Main, Bill was active in a number of local, state, and national professional and service organizations. As with Mayor Furbee, he successfully increased the tax base of his community and greatly expanded the infrastructure of the city.

Both Emerson Van Romig and his son, Richard E. Romig, served as mayors of Keyser. Emerson was a charter member of the Keyser Rotary Club and the WVPA, and served as president of both organizations. Richard served as a commissioned officer and pilot in the United States Army Air Corps during World War II. After the war, Richard held membership in the Nancy Hanks Post 3518, Veterans of Foreign Wars in Keyser. In addition to serving on the board of directors of The National Bank of Keyser, he was active in the Davis Lodge 51, AF&AM, York Rite Bodies, Osiris Shrine Temple, and the Temple of Wheeling. A hunting enthusiast, he was active in the Waco Gun Club. Although remembered as a very popular mayor, records of his administration were unavailable. Despite being a Rotarian, he was sponsored by the Keyser Kiwanis Club for the 1958 Keyser Citizen of the Year Award, an award given by the Kiwanis. In total, the father and son owned Romig's Drug Store for 84 consecutive years from 1899 – 1983.[8]

Richard E. Romig, Jr., relates an anecdote his father used to tell about a moonshiner who would appear at the rear of his pharmacy each Christmas with a gallon of freshly made moonshine to pay his drug bill. Not wanting to offend the 'mountain-man,' Romig would accept the "gift" and credit the man's account with $5.00, which was a fairly significant sum of money in the 1950s. He would then dispose of the potent, distasteful liquid rather than drink it.[9] Richard E. Romig died June 27, 1983 at age 65.

Although a resident and mayor of Bethlehem, Ohio County, West Virginia, Donald C. Sinclair was elected president of the Wheeling Kiwanis Club and was a member of the Wheeling Junior Chamber of Commerce. He was president of the Little Theatre in Wheeling where some considered him "an actor of note." When Sabin vaccine first became available, he organized "Sabin Sunday in Ohio County," a regional drive promoting polio vaccination. He personally prepared and administered the vaccine and helped accomplish the goal of mass immunization against this deadly disease.[3]

James L. Turner was never confronted by an opportunity or challenge that wasn't completed with excellence. He accepted an appointment as pharmaceutical consultant to Fairmont Emergency Hospital, referred to locally as "the state hospital," which was devoted to treatment of alcoholism, drug abuse, and the critically ill under-privileged population of Marion County, West Virginia. He provided a level of care never before experienced at that institution. According to his wife, Mary, "Jim had a problem. He didn't know how to say no!" After receiving encouragement from his pharmacy's patients as well as professional colleagues, Jim Turner somewhat reluctantly filed to run for mayor of Fairmont. His pharmacy kept him quite busy during the day, leaving him little time for other pursuits. After he was elected, a policeman would bring the mail from the mayor's office to his home where he conducted the administrative functions of Fairmont's government at night.[10]

However, Jim's quest for knowledge was unfulfilled by community pharmacy

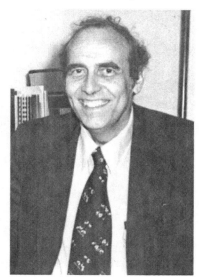

James L. Turner

27

practice. He enrolled in graduate school at West Virginia University
to pursue a graduate degree in pharmacology. He achieved his goal
and received a Master of Science degree in 1964 and a Ph.D. degree in
pharmacology in 1976 to enhance his ability to care for his patients in Marion
County. Jim served as president of the Marion County Pharmaceutical
Association in 1956 and was president of the West Virginia University
School of Pharmacy Alumni Association in 1957.

Four pharmacist-mayors assumed leadership roles at the highest level
of their political party. These leaders, along with their party affiliation and
accomplishments, are noted in Table 1. Four of the 17 pharmacist-mayors
also served on the Board of Directors of a financial institution (Table 2).
Table 3 depicts 10 of these pharmacist-mayors and the honors they received
through their years of public service. Multiple awards from a variety of
sources were not uncommon. This is also not unexpected since pharmacists
have been voted one of the most trusted professionals, and winning the
public's trust and respect is mandatory for civic engagement. Likewise,
patriotism was not lacking in the pharmacists who served as mayor. Seven
pharmacist-mayors served in the armed services during World War I or World
War II, two as commissioned officers. Another who was too old for military
service held a presidential appointment to the War Manpower Commission
during World War II.

Not to be overlooked was the influence of religion on the lives of these
pharmacist-mayors. Fifteen of the 17 were Protestant and two were Catholic.

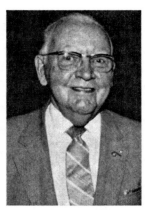
William S. Coleman

All were active members of their respective
churches, with religion being a major factor in the
lives of seven of these individuals. William Sidney
Coleman served both as Deacon and Elder in his
Presbyterian church in Lewisburg and was church
treasurer for many years. Interestingly, Lloyd
Courtney, the church's minister, had practiced
pharmacy prior to entering the ministry. Bill was
very active in the WVPA and rarely missed an
annual convention. Frequently, he was asked to give
an invocation. This occurred with such regularity
that he developed the habit of carrying a prayer
card in his suit pocket. Elwood Bare, mayor of Ronceverte, West Virginia,
obliged virtually every leadership role of the Ronceverte Christian Church.
Donald Sinclair served the Methodist Church as a lay minister through his

years of pharmacy practice. William J. Plyburn chaired the Kuhn Memorial Presbyterian Church Board of Deacons and Elders. Lydia Main is a member of St. Zita's Catholic Church and has served as president of both the Parish Council and of the Altar and Rosary Society. Charles W. Blissitt, mayor of Morgantown, West Virginia, was Superintendent of the Senior Young Peoples' Department of the Wesley Methodist Church from 1960 to 1962. He was also a member of the Wesley Foundation Board of Directors and chaired the Wesley Methodist Church Public Relations Committee. Emerson Van Romig and his son, Richard E., were active in the Keyser Presbyterian Church.

How effective were these pharmacist-mayors during their tenure in office? Three specific examples follow. When Donald Sinclair was first elected mayor, the town treasury had a balance of $23,000 and the police department had only one cruiser that was in poor condition. When he left office, the treasury balance had increased six-fold. New water and sewage systems had been installed, the police department had a fleet of four new cruisers, and each member of the police department was certified by the West Virginia State Police Academy. Taking growth into account, the state designated Bethlehem a city at that time rather than a town. During his tenure, Bethlehem was twice named the most fiscally sound city in West Virginia.[3]

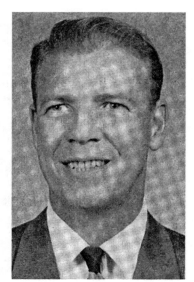

Carl E. Furbee

Following retirement from pharmacy practice and the death of his wife from cancer, Carl Furbee ran for mayor of Bridgeport in 1989 and served eight years as its "full time mayor." His tenure as mayor was extraordinarily productive. He instituted the city manager form of government, obtained funds to build a new fire department facility, and acquired a larger city building. Land was obtained for a proposed city park, and a bridge to the park site was constructed. Carl was instrumental in annexation of the land around the current FBI Fingerprint Division and the local municipal airport, which significantly increased the Bridgeport city tax base, and oversaw construction of the infrastructure (sewage and water) for the FBI facility. Additionally, as mayor he annexed land for the future site of United Hospital Center as well as the Briarwood subdivision with approximately 70 homes. He was instrumental in the development of the South Hills and Shearwood Forest housing subdivisions, as well as the area around the airport where Pratt and Whitney Engine Services, Aurora Flight Sciences and other commercial enterprises have located.[11] As a result of his leadership, the tax base of Bridgeport doubled during Carl Furbee's second tenure as mayor.[12] He ran unopposed in the 1993 and 1995 elections. Mayor Furbee died December 1, 1998, a year after completing his fifth term as mayor.

When Bill Plyburn became mayor of Barboursville, he found a degree of animosity existed between the residents of Barboursville and its sister city of Huntington. Barboursville and Huntington share a common border, making it difficult to determine where one city ends and the other begins. Huntington has a beautiful municipal park called Ritter Park. Barboursville had neither a park nor could it afford one. Mayor Plyburn made acquisition of a park the highest priority of his administration, with a goal of engendering pride in his community. Paul Turman, Sr., Barboursville's current mayor,[13] recalled Bill Plyburn's role in the acquisition of a park as follows: Land for a park had previously been obtained by a former mayor, but it existed as an unsightly, weed-infested field. Bill Turman, a civil engineer who was also city engineer, was a strong proponent of a park and confident he could build one. Together, the "three Bills" devised a plan to build a park yet stay within the city's limited budget. Additionally, demonstrating an element of "one-upmanship," they decided to incorporate a lake in the Barboursville Park and thus surpass Ritter Park. Before long a 70-acre park was constructed with a 17-acre lake as its focal point, surrounded by walking paths and other amenities appropriate for their community. The "three Bills" were rightly proud of their accomplishment. But what should they name the lake? To them, the decision was obvious. They would name it for themselves and call it "Lake William." Thus, Barboursville today has one of the largest man-made lakes in the state of West Virginia, a credit to the "three Bills." [14]

Early in Mayor Plyburn's administration, the development of a mall was proposed for the area. The city of Huntington opposed a mall, fearing the consequences of competition for its downtown stores. However, Barboursville, with a scant business district, had nothing to lose and much to gain. Bill was eager to obtain the mall. Although the mall, developed with 120 stores, is named the Huntington Mall for the more populous sister city, it is located within the municipal limits of Barboursville. When the mall became a reality, it greatly enhanced the Barboursville tax base.[15]

Although some information could be obtained for the pharmacist-mayors who served in the recent past and are well remembered by their constituents, it is impossible to evaluate those mayors who served four or more decades ago. However, a potential gauge of competence is the number of times they were reelected, even though such a measure may be unfair to the mayor who lacked desire to serve multiple terms. Most West Virginia municipalities hold their elections biennially for a two-year term of office. Six mayors were elected twice and four chose to serve a single term. However, six were elected multiple times, for three, four, five, six, 10 and 16 elections respectively. Only one pharmacist-mayor was removed from office and that was due to a legal technicality for living outside the city limits.[9]

Thus, although documented accomplishments for many of the mayors are lacking, it appears that most pharmacist-mayors were both popular in office and successful in accomplishing their goals.

The West Virginia pharmacist-mayors are not without their colorful moments and bits of interesting trivia. George Rice, elected mayor of Shinnston in 1962, entered West Virginia University College of Pharmacy in 1939 and bought the Johnson Drug Store before completing his pharmacy education in 1943. However, by 1946, a dilemma existed. Although three years had elapsed since leaving pharmacy school, George had not been permitted to graduate nor take the state board examination because of failure to take a one class examination from then Dean J. Lester Hayman. By this time, George and his wife were expecting their third child, he owned his own drug store, and was practicing pharmacy, albeit without a license. At Professor Bergy's insistence, he appeared before the dean and was given an oral examination. It has been said Dean Hayman asked one question that George correctly answered. The dean then certified George Rice to be board eligible. He passed the Board of Pharmacy examination February 19, 1946, and became licensed four months prior to receiving his Bachelor of Science in Pharmacy degree that summer.[15]

Rice felt a great sense of responsibility to his community and was best known as a man with a profound depth of civic pride. When Shinnston was struck by a tornado at 8:31 PM on June 23, 1944, he kept the pharmacy open through the night to provide dressings, medications, and sundries necessitated by the disaster. He established a morgue in the basement of a church, set up two aid stations in the town, recruited about 150 men to clear rubble from the two major roadways from the town to facilitate ambulance egress, and went house to house seeking injured people. The following year he and fellow pharmacist, Arch Tetrick, were featured in an *American Druggist* magazine article that recognized them for outstanding community service. In part their citations read, "…his fellow citizens, having testified to his unusual and unselfish activities in behalf of his community, this national citation is made in recognition of his public service as a civic leader and pharmacist." That fall, the Shinnston Business and Professional Club likewise honored both pharmacists. The storm and recognition program were vividly described in a book subsequently published on the subject.[16]

Although George Rice was considered by some to be idiosyncratic, he promoted community pride as exemplified by a personal commitment to neat and clean city streets and sidewalks. He owned a large janitorial brush and swept the streets and sidewalks of Shinnston daily as mayor and in his later years for exercise.[17, 18] George Rice retired from the practice of pharmacy in 1984. At his death on December 28, 2000, a local resident tied a large red ribbon to a janitor's brush and displayed it among the flowers at his funeral.

Dr. Charles W. Blissitt joined the WVU School of Pharmacy faculty as his first job after receiving his doctorate from Mercer University's Southern College of Pharmacy in 1958. In 1960, he was elected to the Morgantown City Council. Two years later he was elected mayor on the first ballot, a week after three attempts to reach a consensus had failed. The opponent he defeated was a three-term mayor of Morgantown.[19] Aggressive both in politics and academia, Blissitt resigned his positions as assistant professor and mayor on July 1, 1964, to accept an appointment as dean at St. Louis (Missouri) College of Pharmacy.[20] In 1970, Blissitt was named dean at the University of Oklahoma College of Pharmacy, a position he held for seven years. After leaving the University of Oklahoma, it is unclear what happened to him. He was last seen at Dillard's Department Store in Austin, Texas, in 2002 selling shoes; certainly, Dr. Blissitt's career has had interesting twists and turns.

Al Carolla, a 1980 graduate of WVU School of Pharmacy and former mayor of Bradshaw, West Virginia (est. pop. 263), has been a volunteer fireman since 1989. Al wanted to be mayor, but once elected he was not enamored with the job. He became an emergency responder and fireman and loved the challenge. Today he serves on the Bradshaw city council and has been with the fire department for seventeen years. [21] Al is West Virginia's only pharmacist-mayor with such an interesting avocation.

West Virginia's pharmacist-mayors were energetic individuals with a strong sense of civic pride, community service, and professional participation. Although they lived in diverse times and in different geographical areas of the state, they shared a caring attitude and the personal and professional attributes that a public servant should possess.

Table 1

Pharmacist-Mayor Participation
at Top Level of District Political Party

Name of leader	Party affiliation	District leadership role
Fred C. Allen	Democrat	Executive committee
Carl E. Furbee	Republican	Executive committee
James L. Turner	Republican	Executive committee
Lydia D. Main	Democrat	Party secretary - treasurer

Table 2

Pharmacist-Mayor Service on Boards
of Directors of Financial Institutions

Mayor	Financial Institution
Fred C. Allen	First National Bank in Marlinton
S. Elwood Bare	First National Bank of Ronceverte
Samuel G. Kapourales	First National Bank of Williamson First Bank of Charleston
Richard E. Romig, Sr.	The National Bank of Keyser

Table 3

Honors Bestowed on Pharmacist - Mayors by Hometowns, Service Clubs, Professional Associations, or Universities

Mayors	City	Honor(s)
Fred C. Allen	Marlinton	Dr. James H. Beal Award Life Membership in WVPA Honorary President of NABP
S. Elwood Bare	Ronceverte	Citizen of the Year 1996
William Sidney Coleman	Lewisburg	Dr. James H. Beal Award Life Membership in WVPA Bowl of Hygeia Award
Carl E. Furbee	Bridgeport	Michael Benedum Fellow Bowl of Hygeia Award Outstanding Alumnus Award of WVU School of Pharmacy
George Karos	Martinsburg	WVU School of Pharmacy Honorary Alumnus Award Bowl of Hygeia Award Sam Walton Leadership Award for Service to Customer Who's Who in WV Business by WV State Journal
Lydia D. Main	Masontown	2000 Pharmacist of the Year Award by Preston County Chamber of Commerce West Virginia Mayor of the Year Award 1996-1997 Bowl of Hygeia Award
William J. Plyburn	Barboursville	Bowl of Hygeia Award
Samuel Kapourales	Williamson	Bowl of Hygeia Award
Richard E. Romig, Sr.	Keyser	Citizen of the Year 1958 by Keyser Kiwanis Club
Charles W. Blissitt	Morgantown	Young Man of the Year Award 1963 by Morgantown Junior Chamber of Commerce

Chapter Four
State Leaders
and Legislators

Pharmacists, as a result of their knowledge, experience and professional service, provide the legislature with a dimension that might otherwise be lacking in non-health care provider public servants. Through the years, a number of pharmacists have distinguished themselves in the West Virginia legislature. Although records are incomplete, pharmacists known to have served in the West Virginia House of Delegates include Clyde W. Fuller, Charles E. Lohr, Robert K. Flanagan, Larry Border and Don Perdue. Delegates Border and Perdue are still serving in 2008.

Three prominent pharmacists with diverse and interesting backgrounds have also served in the West Virginia State Senate. The first pharmacist to

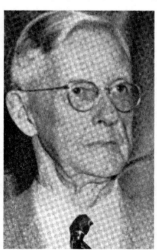

G. O. Young, Courtesy,
West Virginia Pharmacist

be elected a West Virginia state senator was G.O. Young, born in Fairmont, West Virginia, on December 26, 1873 (also see Chapters 10 and 11). Educated with a home study course and an apprenticeship, he was also supposedly the youngest pharmacist ever to be licensed in West Virginia. Throughout his life, his friends and patients knew him by the initials "G.O.," which he preferred to his given name, which was George Orville. G.O. was an outdoorsman who enjoyed hunting and fishing and was a staunch promoter of Mountain State tourism and wildlife sports; as such, he was decades ahead of his time. He traveled through much of the United States, Canada, and Alaska. One of his trips to Alaska beyond the Arctic Circle was described in a book he authored, *Alaskan Trophies Won and Lost.*[1] G.O. was a founder of the West Virginia Chamber of Commerce and in 1921, was named the first chairman of the West Virginia Game and Fish Commission, now the West Virginia

Conservation Commission.[2] G.O. Young was elected state senator for the 15th District of West Virginia in 1934, served three four-year terms and was minority leader during the 1941 and 1943 sessions. He was the 1951 WVPA Beal Award recipient.

Another pharmacist-legislator who served as a West Virginia state senator was Fred Clay Allen. Known to his constituents as "Fred" or "Fred C," he was born on April 18, 1888, in Lima, Tyler County, West Virginia. After high

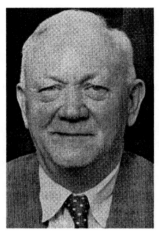

*Fred C. Allen,
Courtesy West Virginia
Pharmacist*

school, Fred enrolled in Valparaiso University College of Pharmacy in Indiana, and received a Ph. G. degree in 1909. During World War I, Fred served in France in the 80th Infantry Division, participating in the Somme Offensive and Meuse-Argonne Campaign.[3] After the war, he returned to civilian life and purchased the Royal Drug Store in Marlinton that he subsequently operated for four decades.[4] Fred kept busy back home: he joined the Episcopal Church, the WVPA, the American Legion, the Elks, the Masonic Lodge, the Shriners, and became active in the Democratic Party. After becoming established in his pharmacy practice, Fred turned his attention to politics and in 1928, ran for mayor of Marlinton. Winning that election, he served the city of Marlinton four years as mayor.

A year after leaving the mayor's office, Republican Governor William G. Conley appointed Fred to the West Virginia State Board of Pharmacy. Fred served with distinction as both a member and president of the Board of Pharmacy for 34 years. Fred's third venture into the political realm began with his decision to run for president of the WVPA in 1934. His confidence bolstered by his previous political successes, Fred entered the 1936 Democratic Party primary for state senator in the 10th senatorial district. Fred had a staunch supporter in Calvin W. Price, Editor of *The Pocahontas Times*, who on March 12, 1936, wrote, "In the generation or more this district has been in existence each of the other counties [of the district] has had the honor of having native sons represent us in the upper house of the legislature, with the single exception of the county on the sunny side of the mountain, our own Pocahontas.. ..This year it looks like our luck has changed. We have no senator seeking reelection. Our candidate, Dr.[a]Allen, was the runner up in

[a] *A title confirmed by the editor of the Pocahontas Times*

the primary four years ago, and came through a close second. No man in the district is more widely and favorably known. He is worthy and fully qualified for the high office."[5] The voters were also told Fred was an environmentalist who loved to hunt and fish, that the economy of Pocahontas County depended on agriculture, and that "Dr. Allen, having been reared on a farm...would stand up for Pocahontas People in the legislature and they would not put anything over on him."[6] After winning the Democratic Party Primary in May 1936, Fred ran unopposed in the general election that fall and subsequently ran unopposed for reelection in 1940 and 1948. In his political career,[b] Fred served the people of Pocahontas County in three capacities: as a West Virginia state senator from 1937 to 1956; on the Democratic Party Executive Committee for more than 20 years; and as Pocahontas County Democratic Party chairman from 1957 to 1960.[7] Retiring from politics in 1960, he thenceforth devoted his time to the profession of pharmacy by continuing to serve on the WV Board of Pharmacy until June 30, 1967. For his years of service to West Virginia and the WVPA, Fred Allen was named the 1955 recipient of the Dr. James Hartley Beal Award. His greatest honor, however, was being named Honorary President of the National Association of Boards of Pharmacy (NABP) in 1958, the only West Virginian to ever achieve this distinction. Fred's service on

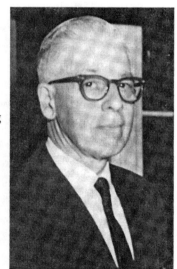

the board came at a time of great change in professional pharmacy licensing. The NABP adopted the four-year baccalaureate degree as the standard for licensure the year Fred joined the WV Board of Pharmacy. That year, the NABP also recognized a need for an accrediting body for pharmacy schools and the American Council on Pharmaceutical Education, now the Accreditation Council for Pharmacy Education (ACPE), was formed. Fred was a proponent of developing a national pharmacy (licensure) examination to replace individual state board examinations, although this did not become a reality during Fred's lifetime. Fred Allen died December 20, 1969, at the age of 81.

The career of a third West Virginia

Herbert Traubert
Courtesy, West Virginia
Pharmacist

---

[b] *According to the editor of the Pocahontas Times, Fred Allen was quite shy and frequently was asked to speak louder to be heard on the Senate floor.*

pharmacist-legislator, State Senator Charles Herbert Traubert, is particularly notable. Born in Wellsburg, West Virginia, on November 11, 1907,[8] Herb enrolled in the WVU College of Pharmacy following high school, receiving a Ph. C. degree in 1929. After graduation, he accepted a position as a staff pharmacist with the Hoge-Davis chain in Wheeling, West Virginia, which he left in 1937 when his father, the sheriff of Brooke County, appointed him deputy sheriff. Herb excelled as a community activist and businessman, and he was revered as an exemplary public servant. However, in large part his reputation was initially established as the sheriff of Brooke County.

Herb's father Joseph Leo Traubert, a baker by trade, was elected sheriff in 1936, but died within a year of assuming office. During his brief tenure, Leo (as he was called) built a solid reputation for honesty, integrity, and fairness. He appointed his pharmacist son, Herbert, "tax-deputy" and put him to work collecting taxes. Little did young Herb know at the time that collecting taxes would be a fateful decision that would thereafter change his life. Before long, the son shared the father's example for exemplary character traits. He was well known at the Brooke County Court and, when his father died, two former sheriffs and a previously defeated sheriff-candidate stepped forward to seek the position.[9] Instead, the court appointed Herb to fill the balance of his father's term. According to an account published in the county newspaper, Herb had been "a most valuable assistant, and it has been many years since the [Sheriff's] office [has] enjoyed or commanded so much respect."[10] A court appointment followed within days and on November 5, 1940, he was elected to a four-year term of his own.

Herb Traubert served Brooke County as sheriff from 1937 to 1945. One morning, Herb and a deputy were driving south on a nearby road in an unmarked patrol car when two hitchhikers solicited a ride. Without identifying himself, Herb asked the pair what they were doing in Wellsburg. One hitchhiker replied they had cigarettes for sale at 50 cents a carton. Knowing something was amiss with a price that low, Sheriff Traubert and the deputy promptly drove the men to the sheriff's office where the hitchhikers confessed to robbing a Wheeling warehouse. About 300 cartons of cigarettes were recovered. By noon, the sheriff and his deputy had the ringleader and four suspects in custody.[11] The men were subsequently convicted and Herb achieved local fame in the "great cigarette caper."

As sheriff, Herb made significant changes in the care of prisoners. The county allotted only 43 cents a day to feed a prisoner. Herb knew a prisoner could not be fed for such a paltry sum. Thus, during his term the standards for incarceration were revised, drunks were driven home, fines were increased as jail occupancy declined, and the quality of the food improved. Financial records of the sheriff's office are no longer available, but a newspaper article of the day predicted this frugal sheriff would have a surplus of funds by the end of his term.[10]

Just as science and technology advanced the pharmacy profession, Sheriff Traubert likewise enhanced the technology available to his office. He was accepted into the FBI National Police Academy and graduated in April 1943. With classmates representing police departments from cities such as Atlanta, New York City, Peoria, and Cleveland, Herb was "right up there with the big boys." On return home, fingerprint technology was introduced to Brooke County and the special agent of the FBI for the Northern (WV) Panhandle thereafter frequented the Brooke County sheriff's office. Patrol cars were equipped with two-way radios for communication with the sheriff's office, the jail, and the police departments of other cities in the Northern Panhandle as well as with other law enforcement offices throughout the region.[11]

Herb left the sheriff's office on July 1, 1945. Although satisfied with his role as sheriff, it was time to return to his chosen profession, pharmacy. With the demands of being a sheriff, he had been unable to practice pharmacy on a regular basis but continued to practice as a relief pharmacist for the Hoge Davis chain to meet the board requirements for relicensure.[12] Now that he was no longer sheriff, it was an ideal time to become a pharmacy owner. In the summer of 1945, Herb purchased Krager Drug Company in Follansbee and renamed it Traubert Drug Company. Herb then purchased the Cove Valley Drug Store in Follansbee in partnership with pharmacist Fred Burnhart, and some months later bought a former candy shop in Hooverson Heights that he converted to a pharmacy. Jimmy Hood, hired as the pharmacist to run that store, later purchased Traubert Drug Company from Herb and renamed it the Hood Drug Company.[12] Thus, in a span of three years the pharmacist-sheriff had become a pharmacist-sheriff-entrepreneur, and his thoughts now turned again to politics and the West Virginia state senate.

The Follansbee Review announced the aspiration of former Sheriff Traubert to enter the West Virginia Senate Democratic primary race to represent Brooke, Hancock, and Ohio counties.[13] Little is known of the basis for Traubert's decision to enter this race, but it probably originated within the Democratic Party headquarters in Wheeling. Without doubt, he had wide support in Brooke County from his successes as sheriff and solid support from the press in Wheeling and Steubenville, Ohio. *The Follansbee Review* clearly championed the candidacy of Herb Traubert as senator by stating his qualifications and emphasizing his pharmacy education. In addition to summarizing his service as sheriff, *The Review* provided a glowing description of Herb's newly remodeled pharmacy, innovations in merchandising, and civic activities, closing with a statement regarding his "fine character" (emphasis added by author) and how, as state senator, he would be a credit to his district.[13] When Herb's grandfather died, the obituary in *The Follansbee Review* prominently made reference to "the family's character" as "upright and honored citizens." [14] Even Herb's dog became known to citizens of Brooke County. When Pat, Herb's white Boston terrier died, an obituary was published in *The Follansbee Review* that was a thinly disguised testimonial to Herb's love for dogs.[15]

After his successful election in 1948, Herb got off to a running start as state senator. Senate President Ralph J. Beam of Moorefield appointed him to four of the most prestigious and powerful senate committees, the Rules, Finance, Judiciary, and Education committees.[16] Beam's appointments were undoubtedly a result of Herb's service as Beam's campaign manager for senate president. Herb did not wait long to introduce bills to be considered for new legislation. In the 1940s, the West Virginia constitution declared, "criminal juries shall be comprised of 12 men," which was interpreted by the attorney general as a proscription for women to serve on juries. In the first week of the legislative session, Herb introduced a proposal for a constitution amendment to permit women to serve on juries in criminal cases. However, the proposed amendment failed, as had one in the previous legislative session. Herb also introduced a bill advocating a statute of limitations on collection of taxes due the state, and another relating to the training of dogs and certain game animals. He supported a World War II veteran's bonus bill. All three of these bills passed and were signed into law.[17] Herb and the other 66 Democrats in the senate voted for a pay raise for secondary school teachers. Unfortunately, Herb was one of only two Democrats who voted for the appropriation bill to fund that pay raise. Thus, it was subsequently defeated. A bill permitting a sheriff to succeed himself, rather than have service limited to a single term, failed to be reported out of committee. In sum, Herb proved to be an active and masterful politician. Although disappointed with the failure of the sheriff succession bill, in a single four-year term he had built a constituency of women, hunters, dog lovers, teachers, and veterans, a worthy beginning for a future legislative leader.

At that time, West Virginia was one of only four states with a two-year school of medicine.[18] To complete their medical education, students traveled to nearby states but many of those graduates settled elsewhere. In fact, only one of every seven medical students who left West Virginia returned, resulting in a dearth of physicians (only one per 1,400 state residents). Then Governor Okey L. Patteson vowed to correct this problem. On January 16, 1951, he made an impassioned plea to the legislature to pass House Bill 477 that would establish four-year programs in medicine, dentistry and nursing.[19] Citing

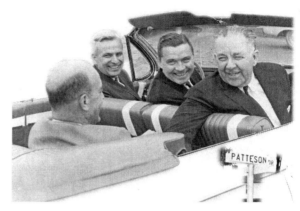

Gov. Okey Patteson (right) with
WVU President Elvis Star, Circa 1960

statistics, the Governor pointed to empty beds in the Veterans Administration Hospitals in Beckley and Clarksburg and a closed wing in the Huntington veterans' facility due to a lack of staff physicians. He suggested the federal government would provide grants to states that initiated action to correct the physician shortage and introduced House Bill 268 to provide funding for the medical school financed with a one-cent tax on soft drinks (the so-called "Pop Tax").[20] As a result of the Governor's plea, the two bills were introduced and were strongly supported by Senator Traubert. However, locating the medical school in Morgantown as Governor Patteson proposed was controversial. The legislators lacked the courage to decide the location and insisted the Governor make the determination. Politicians from Charleston and Huntington wanted the medical school in their hometowns for economic reasons. Politicians from Morgantown also wanted the school in their city due to economic conditions plus they shared Governor Patteson's concern about dismembering the University. The Governor carefully compared each location and over a six-month period consulted with experts around the nation. The experts agreed with Governor Patteson's concerns about harming West Virginia University and in June, 1951, the Governor announced his decision to select Morgantown for financial and academic considerations.[21] Once his decision was announced, politicians from southern West Virginia set out to politically destroy Patteson. After completing his tenure as governor, Patteson retired from the public arena.

Herb was reelected to a second four-year term in the West Virginia State Senate in 1952.[22] Again he managed the campaign of Ralph Beam for senate president and succeeded in helping to get Beam reelected. In turn, Beam reappointed Herb to the same politically powerful committees. However, this time Herb would face new challenges.

The 1953 session of the senate opened with the introduction of a new state aid plan to finance public schools. Prepared by the Joint Committee on Government and Finance and the Commission on Interstate Cooperation, this bill was touted to the press as the most vital issue before the legislature that year. However, on careful reading, Senator Traubert realized this bill was merely a diversion of funds for public school education from the more populous counties of the state to those in northern West Virginia, particularly those counties in the Northern Panhandle.[23] In response, Herb introduced a bill of his own that was more equitable,[24] and through astute political maneuvering he was able to garner the support needed to defeat the funding allocation change.

Only a year elapsed before the next challenge arose for Senator Traubert. This was an impending disaster involving a possible loss of Brooke County's major employer, the Follansbee Steel Corporation, in operation since the early 1800s. A 30 year-old promoter from New York, Frederick W. Richmond, was about to gain control over the publicly owned steel plant, dismantle it, and sell its assets to the Republic Steel Corporation. Republic Steel, considering the sale imminent, announced plans to move the plant to Gadsden, Alabama.[24] Follansbee Steel Corporation employed 720 hourly and salaried workers, most of who lived in Brooke County. Additionally, Sheet Metal Specialty, a separate division of Follansbee Steel Corporation, employed 341 steel workers who would lose their jobs if the sales were finalized. In fact, if Brooke County lost the steel plant, every segment of the region's economy would be affected.[25]

What was the impetus for the sale of the steel manufacturing plant? Since the end of World War II the nation's steel supply had exceeded demand and the price of steel plummeted. Most of the principal stockholders in the Follansbee Corporation resided outside West Virginia and lacked interest in Follansbee's economy. For more than two years, the steel mill had been operating at 70% capacity and profits were down. Major shareholders and directors with stock options (also non-West Virginians) wanted to sell, and

Republic Steel, realizing the purchase price to be a bargain, wanted to buy.

In October 1954, Mr. Marcus A. Follansbee, president and namesake of Follansbee Steel Corporation, announced that the corporate directors had accepted an offer from a group headed by Mr. Richmond to sell the corporate assets for about $9,000,000. A merger agreement with three disparate corporations was in the process of being finalized and, once consummated, a new corporate name would be selected. Proxies had been solicited from shareholders, a majority had approved the sale and the Board of Directors had voted to accept the offer. To the citizens of Follansbee, there appeared to be little they could do to reverse this decision.

Recalling the parable of Gulliver and the Lilliputians, a group of interested citizens took action. Calling themselves the Follansbee Civic Committee, six of the seven-member group were shareholders in the corporation and could justly claim an economic interest. The Committee was elected the previous week at a mass community meeting in the Follansbee Council Chambers. Consisting of an attorney, a real estate developer and former Follansbee plant manager, a Presbyterian minister, the local steel workers union president, the assistant superintendent of Brooke County schools, and the publisher of the *Follansbee Review*, with the Follansbee postmaster and a local businessman the elected alternates, the group met with Senator Traubert to plan their strategy.[25]

The Follansbee Civic Committee filed suit in the Federal District Court of Northern West Virginia for an injunction to prevent the proposed sale of corporate assets.[26] Judge Herbert Boreman blocked the sale of Follansbee Steel's assets and the proposed merger with the various corporations. In his opinion, Judge Boreman held that Follansbee officials had concealed from the stockholders the inducements offered to corporate officials by Mr. Richmond, which included financial compensation of the officers and directors by the new corporation and indemnification of any liability the directors might incur from legal action taken by the shareholders. Follansbee officials also failed to advise the stockholders of these inducements when the proxy vote was solicited. Judge Boreman ruled that the latter constituted fraud and was a violation of the Federal Security Exchange Act.[27]

But the case was not yet over. Senator Traubert received a telegram on November 17, 1954, from West Virginia Senator H. M. Kilgore.[26] The telegram indicated that the Anti-Monopoly Subcommittee of the U.S. Senate Judiciary Committee had investigated the proposed sale of the Follansbee Steel Corporation assets and had also met with the Governor of

West Virginia, the State Attorney General, and the attorneys for both sides in the lawsuit. The preliminary conclusion of the Subcommittee was that violation of various provisions of the anti-trust laws might have occurred. Their investigation was continuing and now involved the Attorney General of the United States and the Securities and Exchange Commission. Senator Kilgore opined, "The Follansbee situation is important not only to the people of Follansbee, but apparently has grave implications in terms of its effect on the national economy. It seems to symbolize a growing tendency towards the destruction of small business and a growth of even larger business concentrations and increased monopolistic practices." [27]

When the December 13, 1954, issue of *Time* magazine was published, Follansbee, West Virginia garnered national recognition.[27] In an article entitled, "Santa Comes to Follansbee," it was stated that, "Only hours before its death sentence was to be carried out last week, the little town of Follansbee, W. Va., got a reprieve — and then a full pardon. Follansbee's doom seemed to be sealed by the deal under which Promoter Frederick W. Richmond would buy out the town's major employer, Follansbee Steel Corp., and sell the mill and inventories to Republic Steel Corp. for dismantling and shipment down South." The article went on to describe the stockholder manipulation with fraudulent intent, the valiant action of the Follansbee Civic Committee, of which pharmacist Traubert played a part, and the true hero of the day, Judge Boreman.[28]

On another political level, Senator Traubert's son, Dick, vividly recalls Herb's involvement in the 1960 campaign for President of the United States.[28] By 1960, Herb had served in the West Virginia Senate for 11 years. He had extensive knowledge of the state's demographics and understood the nuances of West Virginia politics. Herb was one of West Virginia's most prominent Catholic Democrats. In 1960, John F. Kennedy was vying against Hubert Humphrey for the Democratic Party nomination and although leading in the polls, Kennedy's lead in the state was rapidly declining. Senator Traubert was convinced that Kennedy, a Catholic, could not win in West Virginia. Religion, for the first time since 1928 (when Al Smith, a Catholic, was also running for President), was a factor in West Virginia politics. Many Protestants were concerned that the Pope would wield undue influence over a Catholic President, and for Kennedy to win the election it was necessary to change this perception. In early February 1960, John F. Kennedy flew into the Wheeling airport accompanied by his brothers Bobby and Ted. They met with Herb to discuss campaign strategy for West Virginia.

Herb explained that West Virginia was a Protestant state with a sparse Catholic population largely clustered in two cities, Charleston and Wheeling. Although he doubted Kennedy could prevail, Herb felt that if Kennedy won in West Virginia he could win other states. Kennedy named Traubert the area campaign manager, a responsibility that Herb undertook with all the vigor he could muster. A dinner was held as a campaign "kick off" at the Weirton Community Center, with an overflow crowd. The dinner was a huge success, and John F. Kennedy shook hands with every person who attended. Herb's wife held a tea for Jackie Kennedy, and Bobby Kennedy maintained a presence in West Virginia until the May primary election that John F. Kennedy ultimately won.[29] The West Virginia primary, considered unimportant to the Democrats in November 1959, had been pivotal in the election of John F. Kennedy. On January 20, 1961, Senator and Mrs. Herbert Traubert attended an Inaugural Ball in Washington at the invitation of the newly inaugurated President of the United States.

With the election over, Herb's attention once again returned to pharmacy. In 1962, newly elected Governor William Wallace "Wally" Barron appointed him to a five year term on the West Virginia State Board of Pharmacy. Both Republican and Democratic governors reappointed Herb, resulting in a total of 25 years of service with distinction to the board. He served as secretary of the West Virginia Board of Pharmacy from 1962 until his death in 1987. In his last year of service on the board, the West Virginia Pharmacists Association awarded him the Dr. James H. Beal Award.

Perhaps Herb's most enduring achievement to the future of pharmacists in West Virginia is the one least documented and nearly unrecognized: the inclusion of the School of Pharmacy[a] as part of the West Virginia University Medical Center. As previously mentioned, Governor Patteson's bill (H.B. 477) created four-year schools of medicine, dentistry, and nursing. Although the four-year School of Pharmacy had existed since 1936, albeit on the WVU main campus in Morgantown, it was not included in Governor Patteson's bill. Senator Traubert had a lingering concern that the School of Pharmacy would remain on the main campus rather than be included in the new Medical Center (now renamed Health Sciences Center). Since the School had functioned academically within the Medical Center, pharmacists were an integral part of the health care system, and the School's physical facilities

---

[a] *The College of Pharmacy became the School of Pharmacy in 1958*

and support systems were funded through the Medical Center budget, Herb rationalized that the School of Pharmacy belonged physically in the same building.[29] Herb's influence with the WVU Board of Governors was successful and the pharmacy school was ultimately moved to the Medical Center's new Basic Sciences Building.

No biography of Herbert Traubert would be complete without mention of the pride and joy of his life, his Tennessee walking horses. Herb traveled around the country exhibiting them, and equestrian experts were known to visit his property to see them.[30] Unfortunately, this aspect of Senator Traubert's life has long been forgotten and additional information is not available. Fittingly, Herb's portrait is proudly displayed in the WVU School of Pharmacy, the only non-faculty member to be so honored, for his efforts on behalf of the School. Charles Herbert Traubert died on December 26, 1987 at age 80.

Chapter Five

Behind the Counter
to the Front Lines

Pharmacists, by virtue of their chosen profession, have always possessed a strong desire to serve their patients and the public. Similar to others in the health care professions, West Virginia pharmacists also responded to the call to serve their country in times of need. There are undoubtedly many stories of unsung bravery, heroism, or innovative problem solving among the West Virginia pharmacists who served in the armed forces throughout our nation's history. Obtaining their stories is often difficult since many pharmacists might not feel their military actions were particularly noteworthy. In addition, some have died prior to recounting their exploits. However, as the following examples illustrate, West Virginia pharmacists have played an important role in our nation's armed forces.

One such pharmacist was Ralph Stevenson. Ralph Stuart Stevenson was 25 years of age when he enrolled in the College of Pharmacy at West Virginia University in 1948, more mature than many of his classmates as a result of his service in the United States 15th Air Force during World War II. As an aerial gunner/ engineer, commonly known as a "ball turret gunner," on B-24 bombers based in Taranto, Italy, he had been promoted to the rank of staff sergeant. Ralph's selection as a gunner was based on body size: he was the only crewmember who could fit into the confined space of a ball turret. Ralph participated in Operation POINTBLANK,[1] the objective of which was to render the German Air Force (Luftwaffe) ineffective by the time the Allied forces invaded France in 1944. This was to be accomplished by destroying as many German planes as possible in the air and on the ground. Ralph

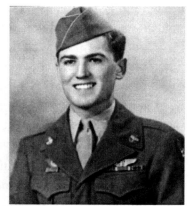

S/Sgt. Ralph Stevenson

flew a total of 35 combat missions over a radius of 500 to 800 air miles from Taranto. Those missions included destroying a large Messerschmitt aircraft complex, shooting down a Messerschmitt 109 fighter and damaging a number of others, bombing a Luftwaffe base in Munich, destroying a ball bearing factory in Steyr, Austria, and bombing the Ploesti oil refineries in Romania where "the sky was filled with German fighters." Bombing raids such as these forced the Germans to decentralize aircraft production to over a thousand small factories, which decreased manufacturing efficiency and disrupted transportation. The success of POINTBLANK saved thousands of lives in the Normandy invasion and hastened the end of the war.

On his bomber group missions, Ralph needed to survive not only German attacks, but also on occasion his own comrades. Pilots arriving from the United States, particularly late in the war, were inexperienced and often poorly trained. On one mission, another B-24 flew directly in front of Ralph's plane. To evade collision, the pilot of Ralph's plane needed to quickly dive from 19,000 feet. It wasn't until they reached 3,000 feet that the pilot could regain altitude and Ralph and his crew could regain their wits.

Ultimately, Ralph's luck ran out during his 35th combat mission on June 13, 1944. His plane was hit by ground fire from anti-aircraft batteries near Innsbruck, Austria. Three of the B-24's four engines were disabled, with failure of the hydraulic and electrical systems. The remaining engine was insufficient to maintain flight speed. Ralph, who had electronics training, was quickly summoned to assess the damage and given its severity, the crew bailed out. At this time, a German Messerschmitt 109 flew up along side. The pilot of Ralph's ship manually lowered the landing gear, an unspoken indication that they were preparing to abandon ship, to which the German pilot waved in response and flew off. Taken prisoner on the ground, Ralph was subsequently held in two prisoner of war camps in Poland and Germany over a period of 11 months.

Ralph's prisoner of war experience was harrowing. The train carrying him to Barth, Germany, packed 50 prisoners in each car and held a total of about 3,000 prisoners of war (POWs). Large letters, POW, were painted on the roof of the cars to prevent allied planes from strafing the train. Only one rest stop was provided for the men to relieve themselves during the five-day trip, resulting in deplorable and unsanitary conditions. Many of the POWs died of dehydration or dysentery en route to their final destination. A fellow prisoner, an American medical officer, provided the only available medical care to the captives.

`On arrival in Germany, Ralph found an overcrowded prisoner of war camp. There were insufficient beds, forcing many prisoners to sleep on the hard, cold floor. Food was almost non-existent and rations consisted largely of Red Cross parcels. Although Hitler had decreed that Air Force captives were to be executed, Ralph's camp commander defied Hitler's order. The cruel alternative, however, was slow starvation. In early February 1945 Red Cross parcels stopped coming altogether. The Germans, running short of rations, consumed the food intended for the prisoners. On the day Ralph was liberated by the Russians at the end of the war, he and his starving comrades observed freight cars loaded with Red Cross parcels they had been denied.

Despite his hardships, Ralph recalled that he was one of the more fortunate prisoners of war. He was one of the relatively few who were transported to prison camp by train, since most POWs were forced to travel across Germany by foot in bitter winter weather conditions. The attrition rate of prisoners forced to march long distances was much greater than those traveling by train, with many succumbing to disease and death along the way.

Following his liberation, Ralph was flown in a B-17 to Reims, France, and from there he was eventually repatriated to the United States. Ralph's 450th Bomber Group received two Presidential Commendations for their outstanding service during World War II. However, his return as a civilian was short-lived. After receiving his pharmacy degree and an ROTC commission, Ralph was ordered to report for active duty and was assigned to the 101st Airborne Infantry Division at Camp Breckenridge, Kentucky. Eventually transferred to the Medical Service Corps as a pharmacist, he rose to the rank of first lieutenant. He was separated from the service September 30, 1952.

Back in civilian life, Ralph initially practiced community pharmacy with Fred Allen in Marlinton, West Virginia, from 1953 to 1957. Ralph later worked as a pharmacist in several small southern West Virginia towns. Eventually he moved to Concord, North Carolina, where he practiced as a pharmacist/manager of a Revco (now CVS) pharmacy for 17 years. Retiring in 1987, he continued to practice as a relief pharmacist until 1995. Ralph is now fully retired and lives in North Carolina.

Another pharmacist who made his mark in the military was John Joseph "Jack" Halki. Jack was a pharmacist and a physician who had two equally prestigious careers in the military and in academic medicine. During World War II, Jack enlisted at age 17 as a Seaman Pharmacist Mate in the U.S. Navy where he commanded an LCM landing craft during his two-

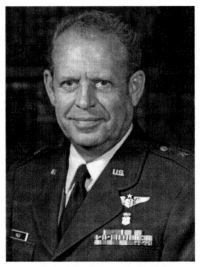

Brigadier General Halki

year enlistment. Although he served in Australia and New Zealand, he did not see combat. Later in his distinguished military career, Jack liked to tell about being found fast asleep in the crow's nest, for which he was reprimanded but not punished. After his return to the U.S., Jack attended West Virginia University and graduated with a Bachelor of Science degree in pharmacy in 1950. Subsequent post-graduate education included an M.D. degree with specialty training in obstetrics and gynecology and a Ph.D. degree in pharmacology (see Appendix B).

Jack entered the U.S. Air Force as a medical officer in 1958, where his assignments varied from flight surgeon to consultant in obstetrics and gynecology to Surgeon General of the U.S. Air Force. He held academic appointments at the University of Texas Health Sciences Center at San Antonio, Texas, and at Wright State University School of Medicine in Dayton, Ohio, before retiring in 1981 from the Air Force with a rank of Brigadier General.[2]

After retiring from the Air Force, Dr. Halki entered academia to chair the Department of Obstetrics and Gynecology as the Nicholas J. Thompson Professor of Obstetrics and Gynecology and assistant dean for Air Force affairs at Wright State University School of Medicine. Dr. Halki retired once again in 1989 to become professor emeritus of both obstetrics and gynecology and pharmacology and toxicology at Wright State University. This retirement lasted 10 years until the president of Wright State University recalled Jack in 1999 to resume the chair of the Department of Obstetrics and Gynecology, a position he held when struck by multiple myeloma.[3]

Although he practiced as a physician throughout his career, Dr. Halki's interest in medications remained in the forefront. His research focus was the study of drugs with abuse potential for the gravid woman and responsible use of drugs during pregnancy. He chaired the Obstetrics and Gynecology Panel for the United States Pharmacopeia (USP) and was a member of the (USP) General Committee of Revision from 1985 to 1990. General John J. Halki was a career military officer, an educator, a clinician, and an exceptional leader in the medical profession. He died of his malignancy on July 29, 2000.

John P. Plummer is an example of a pharmacist who was on active duty in wartime as a line Naval officer. He received a Bachelor of Science degree from the West Virginia University College of Pharmacy in 1943.

Following graduation from pharmacy school, John enlisted in the United States Navy and was commissioned an Ensign. He was assigned as a line officer to a troop transport ship in the Pacific, the U.S.S. Birgit, which unbeknownst to John at the time would eventually become his very own "Love Boat." He became Executive Officer of the Birgit and, by 1946, was Commanding Officer with a rank of Lieutenant

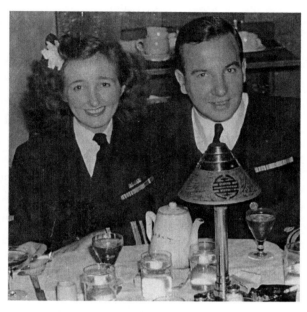

John and Jean Plummer, 1946

Commander. At the end of World War II, the Birgit was assigned to pick up 17 U.S. Navy nurses from the Philippine Islands to be transported to the United States. One of those nurses was Lieutenant Mary Regina "Jean" Garfield from Albany, New York. When the ship arrived in port 11 days later, John and Jean were in love. They subsequently married.[4]

John remained in the naval reserve while practicing pharmacy and retired with the rank of Commander. After return to civilian life, he practiced community pharmacy in Fairmont, West Virginia, where he became owner of an independent pharmacy (also see Chapters 9 and 10). John Patrick Plummer died September 5, 2004, at age 85.

There were a number of pharmacy students over the years whose studies were interrupted by a call to military action. Leo Knowlton is an example of such a student. Leo was born May 23, 1927, in Huntington, West Virginia. He was a senior pharmacy student when the Korean War disrupted his education. He was on active duty in the Marine Corps on two occasions, first during World War II when he served in the continental United States from 1944 to 1946, and again when he served during the Korean War.

Needing tuition money as a pharmacy student in the late 1940s, Leo joined the Marine Corps reserves to help finance his education. On June 25, 1950, eight divisions of the North Korean People's Army crossed the 38th parallel and invaded the Republic of Korea as Leo was enjoying

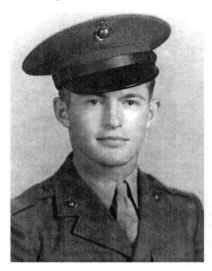

summer vacation prior to his final year in pharmacy school. Within a matter of days, he was recalled to active duty. In vain, Leo wrote a letter requesting a deferment from active duty. Upon receipt of the denial, he stopped by the College of Pharmacy to tell the faculty he had been called to active duty in the Marine Corps. One member of the faculty, Professor Gordon A. Bergy, informed Leo that his son was serving as a medical officer in Korea.

After reporting to active duty, Leo was sent overseas to Japan where they were issued cold weather gear and transported

Sgt. Leo Knowlton

by ship to Wonson, Korea, north of the 38th parallel. On arrival he was assigned to the First Marine Division supply depot at Hungnam, southeast of the Chosan Reservoir. Hungnam had previously been an industrial town with a number of factories; many of the buildings were now damaged and lacked roofs. The Marine Corps utilized these factory buildings as storage depots, with tarpaulins covering the supplies. Hundreds of 55-gallon oil drums were also "stacked high" on the beaches at the seashore for storage.

On November 27, 1950, the communist Chinese struck the Marine positions in force in an attempt to destroy Leo's division. Marguerite Higgins, the famous female war correspondent, later reported the main body of Chinese began infiltrating North Korea on the night of October 14. More than 30 divisions — two Chinese Armies — had amassed by the opening of the offensive.[5] According to Leo, "The Chinese came a whooping and a hollering over the hill, like they were all doped up on heroin or cocaine." Leo was not involved in the actual fighting as his supply unit withdrew ahead of the Chinese onslaught. They withdrew all the way to Masan, the entire length of the Korean peninsula, in what is now known as the Pusan Perimeter. After the withdrawal, "a demolition crew came in and blew up all those supplies to prevent the Chinese from recovering them," Knowlton recalls.

It was at Masan that Knowlton discovered what a truly small world we live in. It turned out that the younger Dr. Gordon G. Bergy was a physician on active duty as a medical officer in the same First Marine Division as Leo. According to Knowlton, he was at the railroad depot when a hospital train came in. Leo decided to start asking officers getting off the train if they knew a Dr. Bergy. After a time, Leo heard a man respond, "I'm Dr. Bergy." Leo introduced himself and explained he was one of his father's pharmacy students and that his father told Leo his son was in Korea as a medical officer. "That sort of helped me when I got back to college," Knowlton explained. Professor Bergy told Leo "his son wrote him and said he had met one of his students over there." Professor Bergy then added, "Leo was a changed man."

After his return to the United States as a sergeant and his completion of pharmacy training, Leo initially worked at an independent community pharmacy. It was here that he met his wife, Betty, on a blind date. Betty had a clerk friend who worked at the pharmacy and arranged the date. According to Leo, "Betty worked at Monsanto in Charleston, West Virginia, at the time. It was a blind date for me but not for her. She knew where I worked, so — unbeknownst to me — she and her mother came into the pharmacy to look me over." For Leo all is not fair in love and war. Over time, he accepted a position as assistant director of pharmacy at the Charleston Area Medical Center and retired in 1987. Since retiring, Leo and his wife have taken 40 cruises and traveled most of the world. Their marriage has endured for 53 years and will hopefully last for several additional cruises. They continue to reside in Cross Lanes, West Virginia.

Clyde Eugene Reed is a World War II combat veteran with a short pharmacy career interspersed between his military service and a career in dentistry. As a youth, Clyde loved music and became proficient as a drum major and French horn player. He was drafted into the U.S. Army in 1942, early in World War II. After receiving basic training in Texas, he arrived in Hawaii by a circuitous route and was assigned to the 27th Infantry Division Band as drum major and French horn player. As a musician he held the technical rank of T-4, equivalent to the rank of sergeant.

The 27th Infantry Division, along with two U.S. Marine Divisions, invaded Saipan in the Mariana Chain of Islands in June 1944. Clyde saw combat for 25 days until the island was taken. Daily patrols were necessary to secure the island. According to Clyde, "the infantry would take one hill or ridge...[and] dig fox holes to protect the gain against counter attacks. In the meantime, the Navy or Air Force would pound the next ridge with everything they had. When the fire was lifted, the infantry would rush the hill and repeat the process."

Clyde's division also had to contend with frequent Banzai attacks in which Japanese stragglers attacked the Americans with bayonets affixed to rifles or poles. These attacks became more frequent after the Japanese had expended their ammunition. On one occasion, Clyde and a buddy were caught in a cave with a Japanese soldier lobbing hand grenades toward its entrance from the hill above. The Japanese women on the island had been taught that the Americans were cruel and would torture them if captured.[7] According to Clyde, when Americans approached them, the women and the children would jump off the cliff to commit suicide rather than surrender to the Americans. During the final phase of operations on Saipan, Clyde was transferred to the hospital to perform medical aid and hospital orderly duties. Clyde thus proved to be the prototypical pharmacist: one who can and, as expected, will do everything.

Following his return to the U.S., Clyde received a Bachelor of Science degree in pharmacy from the West Virginia University College of Pharmacy in 1951. After graduating, he obtained a Doctor of Dental Surgery degree from the University of Maryland School of Dentistry. Clyde practiced dentistry in Baltimore, Maryland, until he retired in 1987. He now resides in Punta Gorda, Florida.

In wartime, loss of life is inevitable and pharmacists are not immune. Four former WVU pharmacy students were killed in action in the European Theatre of Operations during World War II. Of these, two were enlisted men and two were commissioned officers.[8]

Private Robert John Campbell was born December 1, 1913, in Stanford, West Virginia, and operated a Kanawha County food market prior to enrolling in pharmacy school. From a family of modest means, he worked several years to save for a college education. Inducted into the Army before graduation, he was assigned to Company I, 358th Regiment of the 90th Infantry Division in England that was preparing to invade France. Entering Normandy at Utah Beach on June 10, 1944, the division fought through the bocage — ubiquitous hedgerows that partitioned pastures and favored the German defenders — with a mission of cutting off the Cotentin Peninsula and isolating the port city of Cherbourg. The rain began to fall on July 3 and continued each day through the twelfth. Mud was ankle deep, foxholes were filled with water, and the soldiers were soaked to the skin. They hadn't had a hot meal or a shower for two weeks.

From July 8 through July 12, the entire regiment was engaged in a battle to capture a forested hill near the base of the Cotentin Peninsula that overlooked the English Channel. Hand-to-hand fighting had been bitter and the Germans vastly outnumbered the Americans. Casualties in those five days were heavy, totaling 309, with 17 men from the 358th killed in action. However, the 358th won the battle and commanded the surrounding countryside, essential for artillery fire control. A Presidential Unit Citation was awarded to the 3rd battalion for their courage and tenacity in routing the enemy from a seemingly impregnable fortress.

After a night's rest, on July 13 the 358th moved to the southeast and soon encountered strong enemy resistance from the 2nd SS Das Reich Division, Germany's foremost fighting force. By mid-morning, the battalion had gained only 300 yards due to unrelenting enemy machine gun fire. Stiff resistance continued into the afternoon. It was not until 8 PM that Company I entered the village of Gorges, little over a mile from that morning's starting point. Pvt. Campbell was killed that day, one of 79 casualties sustained by the 358th Regiment.[9] Robert was posthumously awarded a Purple Heart medal and the unit was awarded a Presidential Unit Citation.

Another combatant fighting in Normandy was Ralph Raymond Ferguson of Scarbro, West Virginia. Ralph was born February 23, 1920, and he received a Bachelor of Science degree in pharmacy and an infantry commission as Second Lieutenant with the class of 1943.[10] Assigned to Company E, 116th Infantry Regiment of the 29th Infantry Division, he participated unscathed in the invasion at Omaha Beach on D-Day. However, Ralph died of a head wound in the vicinity of St. Clair sur L'Elle six days later on June 12, 1944,[11] not far from where Robert Campbell was to die the next month. Unfortunately, transmitting this information to his family proved to be difficult. Ralph's wife was informed on June 11 by War Department telegram that Ralph had been killed on D-Day (June 6).[12] Then, ironically, Ralph's mother Mrs. Beatrice Ferguson received a letter on July 26, 1944, that her son had written on June 11. Several weeks elapsed before the confusion was corrected. For a family to lose a husband or son is devastating enough, without adding uncertainty to intensify the grief. Ralph was also posthumously awarded a Purple Heart medal.

George Charles Rangos, like Robert Campbell, was drafted before completing his pharmacy education. PFC Rangos of Wellsburg, West Virginia, was born November 7, 1924, and was an honor graduate of the Wellsburg High School class of 1942. George came from a large family with five sisters and two brothers. He enrolled in the WVU College of Pharmacy that fall but was inducted into the Army in May 1944 after completing only two years of the pharmacy program. Assigned to a medical battalion as an aid man, George sustained serious head injuries in February 1945 while treating battlefield casualties in Germany.[13] Evacuated to Camp Picket (Virginia) Hospital, he died of wounds on April 16, 1945.[14] His youngest brother Charles, Jr., recalled the arrival of George's body from Camp Picket. "George had been a popular teen and a record number of the town's people turned out to show their respect." His funeral was held at the family residence on Sunday, April 29, 1945, with military rites at the graveside. Like Robert Campbell and Ralph Ferguson, George was awarded a Purple Heart.

Finally, the story of Army Medical Corps Major Michael A. Rafferty is an interesting, albeit sad tale of a highly educated man with little opportunity to practice his skills. Michael Alfonso Rafferty was born December 24, 1903, in Camden, WV (population then 330). He graduated from St. Patrick's High School in Weston before enrolling in the West Virginia University College of Pharmacy where he received a Ph.C. degree in 1929. Graduating first in his pharmacy school class he received the Lehn and Fink Gold Medal, awarded in honor of his class standing. From 1929 to 1931, he studied biochemistry and pharmacology, earning a Ph.D. at Duquesne University in Pittsburgh. Returning to Morgantown, Michael enrolled in the two-year WVU School of Medicine program, receiving a Bachelor of Science

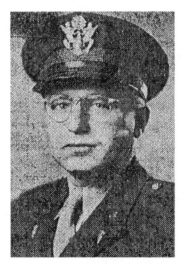

Major Michael A. Rafferty

degree in medicine in 1933. He earned an M.D. degree from Rush Medical College in 1935 and completed a residency in Chicago in June 1937. Once again returning to Morgantown, he joined the medical school faculty where he taught until 1941,[15] at which time he resigned his appointment to accept a research position at Miles Laboratories in Elkhart, Indiana. After the war began, Michael entered the armed services in June 1942 as a Captain in the U.S. Army Medical Corps. Promoted to Major before leaving for overseas duty in February 1944,[16] he was assigned to the M-409th medical supply depot in Liege, Belgium, that supported the First and Ninth Armies. By October 1944, Liege had become a major center for medical supplies arriving from Antwerp. As supply operations for the two armies increased, Liege became a primary target for the German V-weapons [Vergeltungswaffen or Revenge Weapons]. Between November 20 and 30, 1944, Liege was hit directly 230 times with another 1,000 V-1s and V-2s exploding nearby.[17] Major Rafferty was killed on November 24, 1944 during a V-weapon attack on Liege while providing care for wounded from the nearby Huertgen Forest Offensive. He was one of 92 service men killed and 336 wounded in Liege by V-1 attacks between September 1944 and March 1945.[17] He was also posthumously awarded a Purple Heart medal. Major Rafferty died while serving his country, a brilliant man whose life was taken much too soon.

Each West Virginia pharmacist who served with an army ROTC commission in the armed forces during the Korean War served with an infantry commission. ROTC commissions in other branches of the service were not available in the 1940s and the 1950s as they are today. Four West Virginia pharmacists held commissions in that era: one in France with the USAF and three in Korea as infantry officers. Edward Rockis is one of these individuals.

Edward W. Rockis was an outstanding pharmacist, military hero, officer and gentleman. Ed was an all-state fullback at Morgantown High School who also excelled in basketball and track.
He attended West Virginia University College of Pharmacy and graduated in 1951 with a Bachelor of Science degree and ROTC commission as Second Lieutenant in the infantry.

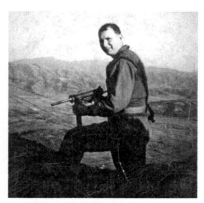

Lt. Ed Rockis in Korea

Ordered to active duty in December 1951, Ed reported to The Infantry School at Ft. Benning, Georgia, where he completed the Associate Infantry Company Officers Course (AICOC) in April 1952. His exceptional leadership skills were recognized at Ft. Benning and Ed was offered the MTC Course for exceptional leaders that he completed in October 1952. Upon arrival in Korea, Ed was assigned to the renowned 15th Infantry Regiment of the Third Infantry Division, in which Generals of the Army George C. Marshall [18] and Dwight D. Eisenhower [19] had also served. Wounded in action on March 19, 1953, Ed was awarded the Purple Heart. Ten days later Ed was promoted to First Lieutenant and was back in action. The following month, he received a wound to the left thigh. Out of action for five weeks to recuperate, he again returned to his unit. In early May, Ed was transferred to Company L. Company L had not performed well in combat and new leadership was deemed necessary. Rockis, a First Lieutenant for only a month, was selected for the position of company commander and transferred to the third battalion.

On the night of June 10-11, 1953, while defending a position, his company was attacked by a large enemy force. Under heavy mortar and artillery fire, Ed moved about the shell torn terrain encouraging his men and coordinating the holding action. However, Ed lost contact with several of his men when communication with a listening post was disrupted by incoming artillery fire and the individuals there were stranded. Lieutenant Rockis bravely led a rescue force through intense mortar and artillery fire to reach the isolated men at the listening post. Finding one man seriously wounded, he administered first aid and carried the wounded man back to the main line of resistance.[20] For gallantry that night, Lt. Rockis was awarded the Silver Star medal.

His executive officer recalled an event of July 16, 1953, and wrote: "The Chinese had broken through a ROK [Republic of Korea] Division, and all units were moved. We were told to occupy a certain hill. It was pouring rain and very dark when we got there. We moved our platoons into defensive positions for the night. Ed and I lay on the ground and finally went to sleep. The next morning we were sitting and talking when we heard a 76 mm artillery shell coming in. They generally fired about three. When the first one hit, we flattened on our stomachs and waited. When the second one came in, I jumped up and ran about five yards and dived behind a rock ledge. The third round came in but it sounded further off. At this time, Ed came crawling around the ledge and told me he was hit. I checked him out, put a bandage on him, and called for a litter bearer. I told him he had a million dollar wound; he would live but was going home. That was the last time I saw him…it was my privilege to have served with him. He was a fine man and an outstanding officer." [21] Ed was awarded a Purple Heart with an Oak Leaf Cluster, indicative of another — his third — Purple Heart.

Ed was separated from active military duty on November 29, 1953. In December 1954, he was honored by the King of Greece for his leadership of Greek troops attached to the Third Division in Korea. The citation read, "For services rendered, a Royal Order to bestow the Medallion Exereton Praxeon (Meritorious Service Medal) to Lieutenant Rockis for having given invaluable service to the Greek Expeditionary Forces in Korea, contributing greatly to the success of the missions undertaken by those forces against an enemy of the United Nations for the defense of world freedom."

Following Ed's return home to Morgantown, he continued to serve his country as a board member of the Selective Service System from 1965 to 1976, for which he received certificates of appreciation from Selective Service Director Lewis B. Hershey and Presidents Richard M. Nixon and Gerald R. Ford.

It is not generally known that Ed Rockis initially wanted to be a veterinarian, but was encouraged to enroll in pharmacy school by his brother-in-law, fellow pharmacist and mentor, Joe Nemeth. His interest in veterinary medicine continued, however, and his independent pharmacy, City Pharmacy in Morgantown, became the center for veterinary pharmacy practice in north central West Virginia. Ed continued to practice pharmacy until September 1988 when he died of complications following surgery.

A pharmacist colleague, classmate, and friend of Ed Rockis, Jim Fredlock, related a close encounter with death that he personally experienced while on active duty in the army during the Korean War. James William Fredlock was born September 17, 1929, in Morgantown, West Virginia. He graduated with the West Virginia University College of Pharmacy class of 1951 with a Bachelor of Science degree and an Infantry ROTC commission as Second Lieutenant. Reporting for active duty at The Infantry School at Ft. Benning, Georgia, in July 1951, he was

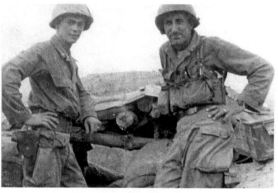

Lt. Fredlock and Sgt. First Class Zimmerman on Pork Chop Hill

ordered to the port of embarkation four months later upon completing the Associate Infantry Company Officers Course.

Upon arrival at Northern Honchu Island, Japan, Jim was assigned to the 24th Infantry Division for weapons and tactical training. From Japan, Jim was sent to Korea where he was assigned to the 179th Regiment of the 45th Infantry Division as a platoon leader in E Company. Jim vividly recalls the night of June 21, 1952, when he received his baptism of fire. A battalion of attacking Chinese overran his position on the south side of Pork Chop

Hill, so named because of its shape. Two thirty caliber heavy machine guns attached to his Second Platoon were knocked out early. According to the after action report, prior to the Chinese attack the Second Platoon received 5,000 rounds of incoming fire.

As the Chinese attacked up the trench line, a "potato masher" grenade exploded in close proximity to Jim's face, knocking his glasses off and throwing him to the ground. As Jim lay on the ground, Chinese troops ran over him with one man removing his wristwatch. He feigned death until the Chinese cleared his position, at which time he called in variable timed (VT) fire on the hill, the timing of the explosions set to be most lethal to the enemy. Two men in his platoon were captured and taken by the Chinese as prisoners of war. In addition to the two captives, the cost of the action in the Second Battalion that night was 29 killed and 130 wounded. As the sun rose the next morning, Lt. Fredlock and the remaining three survivors walked off Pork Chop Hill. Pork Chop Hill frequently changed hands. A favorite story recounted by Lieutenant Fredlock relates to an inebriated soldier from his company at a time the hill was held by the Chinese. Liquor was prohibited when on line, but the soldier somehow acquired some. He removed a Thompson submachine gun from the company command post and crossed a rice paddy to Pork Chop Hill. There he shot three enemy soldiers and returned to his unit. In withdrawing from Pork Chop Hill, he sustained three bullet wounds inflicted by the Chinese. His Company Commander, furious for the rule infraction and needless risk of life, was nonetheless faced with a dilemma: punish the man by courts-martial or reward him with a medal. Ultimately, it was decided that if the wounded man lived, he would be reassigned rather than returned to his former company. Investigation failed to determine the source of the liquor, which remained a mystery for 46 years. Then, in 1998, the 45th Division held a reunion in Oklahoma City, Oklahoma. All the principals of this incident except for the miscreant were there: A Texan nicknamed "Skinny" admitted to the Company Commander (now a retired Colonel) and Lt. Fredlock that he supplied the whiskey to the young soldier. The drunken soldier who perpetrated the incident survived his wounds and served his punishment: banishment from E Company for 46 years.

After the war, Jim returned to Morgantown where he practiced pharmacy with his father for 36 years and eventually owned the pharmacy, aptly named Fredlock's Pharmacy. Currently, Jim is retired and divides his time between Morgantown and Florida.

Douglas Dennis Glover is an example of a pharmacist and a soldier who also became an obstetrician. His father was a community pharmacist who passed along his love of the profession to Doug. Like his two colleagues described previously, Doug graduated from the West Virginia University College of Pharmacy in 1951 with a Bachelor of Science degree and an Infantry ROTC commission as Second Lieutenant. Following graduation, he was ordered to active duty and assigned to The Infantry School at Fort Benning, Georgia, on August 17, 1951.

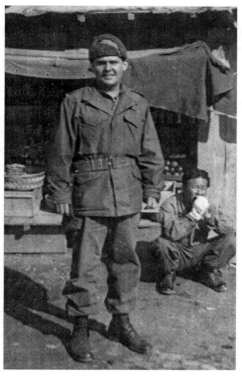

Lt. Glover at an open-air pharmacy in Taejon, Korea, circa 1952

While at Ft. Benning, Doug applied for transfer to the Medical Service Corps as a pharmacist. Pharmacists were not yet commissioned in that era, and a Master Sergeant with hash marks indicating many years of service informed Glover "pharmacists make excellent machine gunners! Forget the transfer, the need is greater in the Infantry." Glover knew better than to argue. However, that sergeant fully understood Glover was no hero and seeking no medals. Thus, orders were received after completion of the AICOC to report to Fort Sam, Houston, Texas, to the Medical Field Service School where Doug enrolled as a student at Brooke Army Medical Center.

Upon arrival in Korea on May 1, 1952, Doug was assigned to the 120th Medical Battalion of the 45th Infantry Division. The 45th Infantry Division was the Oklahoma National Guard division prior to its activation, and Glover was among the earliest "non-Okie" replacements assigned to the division. One of the first individuals he met was Captain Harley Harris, who introduced himself and advised Glover not to bother with his name because Harley was due to return to the "States" any day. Six weeks later, a dejected Harley Harris was still in the division and Glover still didn't know his surname.

Of Glover's military experiences, there is one of which he is particularly proud. In June 1952, the 45th Division pulled back for six weeks of rest for its battle weary troops. Since he hadn't been in combat, Doug didn't warrant a prolonged rest. Instead, he was assigned to establish a triage and medical evacuation unit south of the Punch Bowl near the east coast of Korea. Doug was a young soldier, separated by many miles from the rest of his division, and told to establish a unit by whatever means appropriate. The Punch Bowl was a circular mountain whose shape suggested a large bowl with a high mountain projecting bilaterally to both east and west. The terrain was flat to the south, with a road and a parallel rail line coursing southward out of the artillery range. It was ideally suited for a medical evacuation facility that was greatly needed by the U.S. 40th Infantry Division for evacuation of wounded soldiers to the M.A.S.H units to the rear.

"I was given two ambulance platoons, a rifle platoon, a kitchen unit and two litter jeeps to establish this evacuation unit," Doug recalled. A collecting unit with a receiving tent, where wounded men and medical evacuees were transported by litter jeep, was set up by Glover to the south of the Punch Bowl. A bus fitted with railroad wheels to run on a track with litters in tiers suspended from the ceiling on both sides of the vehicle was also devised, so that eight patients could be evacuated simultaneously. A helicopter was used for immediate air evacuations. Two medical officers were also assigned for triage purposes. Fifty years after its founding, this evacuation unit was still at the same location with the same mission.

Glover also described a situation that tested his leadership ability. Late one afternoon near suppertime, he and some buddies were playing bridge and relaxing in the officers' tent when a knock was heard at the door. Sergeant First Class Zimmerman appeared to inform Glover the cooks were on strike and refused to prepare supper. Emerging from the tent, Glover observed an angry crowd of hungry enlisted men standing in a line rattling their mess gear. Sgt. Zimmerman could give no valid reason for the cooks to strike. Zimmerman, whom Glover highly respected, was a 45th Division National Guardsman with experience dating to the Sicilian and Italian campaigns of World War II. Never had the sergeant been presented with a problem he could not resolve.

Zimmerman and Glover walked to the cook's tent where the cooks were found playing poker. "Tens hut," Sergeant Zimmerman barked, only to be ignored by the cooks. Lieutenant Glover then asked the cooks why they were on strike. The cooks continued playing cards on their bunks. More silence. Addressing the cooks once again, Glover inquired if they had a gripe to discuss, but to no avail. The cooks were directly challenging Glover's authority and felt they had the upper hand; however, they were soon to find out just how good they had it as cooks.

On the way back to the officer's quarters, Glover thought of a solution. He first called Jim Fredlock in the 179th Regiment that was at the front. When asked if Fredlock needed any riflemen, Jim said he would take all he could get. Glover explained he had six belligerent and rebellious men who were a discipline problem that he would like to transfer to a unit at the front. When Fredlock agreed to take them, Glover received approval for a request for transfer. A two and a half ton truck was immediately dispatched. Sergeant Zimmerman stoically ordered the cooks to pack their duffle bags. They were informed of their destination as the truck was pulling out. Some years later when speaking about the incident, Lt. Fredlock recalled that two of the six men were unfortunately killed in action. However, each of the former cooks had performed well with active combat bringing out their best.

Reflecting back on events that occurred in Korea, there was one particularly tragic incident that remained with Glover over the years. As he relates the story, "I don't recall his name. I have managed over the years to push it out of my mind. He arrived as a replacement in the 279th Infantry Regiment mid-winter 1953, a few months before the Panmunjon "peace talks" began. He was young and inexperienced, having just arrived from the states. But he was eager to 'see some action' and volunteered for the first patrol to be formed after his arrival."

"Winters in Korea are cold, particularly if you are located north of the 38th parallel. This night was no exception. The patrol failed to make contact with the enemy and returned just prior to daybreak. En route to Korea, the youth purchased a 45-caliber pistol in Japan that he wore in addition to a carbine he carried. Having had no training with a pistol, he was unaware of the danger created by a round in the chamber. On return to the main line of resistance, he attempted to eject the round from the chamber without success. The slide was frozen and would not move. As he continued to struggle with the slide, the muzzle eventually pointed to his body and he inadvertently pulled the trigger. The bullet entered his body behind the pubic bone and lodged in the pelvis. Numerous attempts to administer plasma failed. His veins had collapsed; he was in shock. He died in my arms. We later learned he was only 17 years old when he died. He had left home at age 15 to enlist in the army but was rejected due to his age. A second attempt to enlist at 16 also failed. Somehow, he succeeded in deceiving the recruiters the third time. Writing that letter to his parents in an attempt to attach some purpose to his death was the most difficult task I had ever undertaken," Glover said.

After returning to civilian status, Glover practiced community pharmacy for four years before entering medical school. He received an M.D. degree from Emory University School of Medicine in 1961. After completing a residency in obstetrics and gynecology, he entered private practice as an obstetrician and gynecologist in Marietta, Georgia, for 17 years, followed by a career in academic medicine for 22 years. Doug is currently professor emeritus of obstetrics and gynecology and pharmacy at West Virginia University in Morgantown.

Ralph Stevenson, Jack Halki, John Plummer, Leo Knowlton, Clyde Reed, Ed Rockis, Jim Fredlock, and Doug Glover represent but a few of the West Virginia pharmacists who distinguished themselves by their military contributions or had a story to share. At least four of their number who served in World War II, along with undoubtedly others from World War I, Viet Nam, or other military conflicts, were less fortunate, having their voices silenced and their careers shortened as a result of combat. This chapter is dedicated to all the West Virginia pharmacists, male and female, who served their country at home or abroad, in war and at peace.

Chapter Six

Heroes

West Virginia is a state prone to natural disaster. Its mountainous terrain, with many rivers, streams, and ample rainfall, contribute to flooding in valleys and low-lying areas. Nine pharmacists in recent years have become heroes due to their actions associated with flash floods or tornados. The stories of these heroic pharmacists and the circumstances contributing to the disasters are told here.

Eight thirty one on the evening of June 23, 1944, is a moment in time most residents of Shinnston will never forget. At that precise minute, the little city of Shinnston was struck by a catastrophic tornado that destroyed their town and took many lives. However, Shinnston was fortunate in having two pharmacists who that night personified the definition of hero: George Rice and Arch Tetrick. From the time the tornado struck to 4:30 AM the next day, George (see Chapter 3) exercised exceptional leadership skills that are rarely found in civilians. He established a morgue, set up and helped staff two aid stations, organized crews to clear highways, and directed evacuation of the injured and critically ill to area hospitals.

Arch was in his pharmacy shortly before the tornado struck when he noted the sign outside "swinging crazily back and forth in the heavy wind."[1] Concerned the sign was about to be torn from its mooring, Arch stepped outside to investigate. The sky was eerily black; an occasional clap of thunder could be heard, accompanied by lightning flashes in the sky. Moments later a man with severe lacerations staggered into his pharmacy seeking medical attention, telling Arch that the Pleasant Hill section of Shinnston had been hit by a tornado with many of the residents lying injured or dying. Arch took the bleeding man to a nearby clinic and asked how he could be of help. Hearing that the clinic needed bandages and first aid provisions, Arch returned to the pharmacy and sent his clerk to deliver the items to the clinic. An aid station was set up in the basement of the Methodist church that was also supplied by Arch. Arch spent the night tirelessly going from one aid station to the other providing narcotics, syringes, bandages, and first aid supplies to those in need. At dawn the next morning, Arch was astonished at the extent of the damage. Debris from demolished homes blocked roads, trees had been uprooted, and cars overturned. Shinnston was unrecognizable, with many areas having been destroyed within minutes.

National recognition for pharmacists Arch Tetrick and George Rice followed in the ensuing months. The two men were featured in the July 1945 issue of *American Druggist.* In September 1945, The Shinnston Business and Professional Men's Club presented a program attended by several state pharmacy dignitaries to honor the two heroes. Both Rice and Tetrick received an *American Druggist* Citation for Outstanding Community Service.[1]

Pharmacist Jim Burks had a harrowing experience with a flood in 1985.[2] Although Marlinton, West Virginia, has experienced several floods over the past two decades, the worst occurred in November 1985. Jim owned his pharmacy for only eleven months when disaster struck. He had attended a Rotary Club meeting earlier that Monday evening. Since it had been raining about three days and he was new in town, Jim was advised to expect two or three inches of water in his store. To prepare for this, Jim returned to the pharmacy and raised everything about waist high. As he left the store, he noticed a group of six or seven senior citizens who needed a ride across town. Jim decided to offer them a lift in his truck, with some riding in the front seat and the rest in the back. At 8:30 PM, Jim passed the confluence of Knapps Creek and the Greenbrier River, near a railroad depot, when the water rose over the doors of his truck. Fortunately, the engine did not stall and Jim was able to deliver the senior citizens, wet and scared but unharmed, to their destination. Given the rapidly rising water, though, Jim decided to leave his truck and returned to town in the bucket of an end loader along with a state policeman and state road worker. At that point, the water was so deep that they rescued people from second story windows as they drove along the route. As they passed Jim's pharmacy at 10 PM, they could see the now floating ice cream freezers striking the pharmacy ceiling. Jim and the others worked tirelessly over the next several hours to move people to safety until the end loader's engine stalled. The group then waded through the water to the second floor of the fire station where they spent the night. Throughout the night, Jim heard house trailers from the mobile home parks being washed over the bridge near town. When dawn broke, Marlinton resembled a war zone. Cars were piled on top of each other, with mud and debris everywhere. "There was no way to get in or out of Marlinton," Jim recalled. "The town was blocked at both ends by water, the Greenbrier River blocking one end and Knapps Creek blocking the other."

Absent a warning about a potential flood and with the firemen frantically working to rescue people, the fire trucks had not been moved to safety. Four fire engines and all the police cars were damaged or destroyed. There was no electric power and no food. It didn't matter at the time that the people had no money since there wasn't anything to buy. Commerce in the valley had come to a complete standstill. The Salvation Army and the American Red Cross arrived in Marlinton the following afternoon to provide food and bottled water. Seven or eight dead victims of the flood were identified.[2] "As a new pharmacy owner, I had insurance but soon found there was no flood coverage," Jim related. "I lost everything in the pharmacy but the clock over the door where the flood water could not reach it. Billie Myers, the other pharmacist in Marlinton who owned Royal Drug, lost his pharmacy as well as his home. Because of his age and poor health, Billie retired from pharmacy practice." However, Jim Burks was committed to the community and felt it was his responsibility to rebuild. Within three days, he opened a temporary pharmacy at the hospital to provide medications to the public. Jim also owned a pharmacy in Durbin, West Virginia, and transferred inventory from Durbin to Marlinton. Although wholesalers were unable to reach the pharmacy to supply medications, he had sufficient inventory to provide patients with needed life-saving drugs until the roads were cleared.

Steve Crawford of Elkins, West Virginia, was director of pharmacy at Davis Memorial Hospital at the time of the 1985 flood. He recalled that the flood left the small towns in that area in desperate need of medical supplies. Emergency medical services' helicopters from the state government flew into Davis Memorial Hospital where they were loaded with essential medications such as antihypertensive drugs and insulin for delivery to the areas in need. They were notified by short wave radio of which drugs were needed. When Steve's supply of pharmaceuticals began to run low, Ben Exley from Clarksburg [Wholesale] Drug Company allowed Steve to drive his pick-up truck to their warehouse to load it with supplies. The wholesaler's warehouse was literally emptied in the process. At one point during the relief efforts, the weather was so bad that Sam Chanel, assistant medical director of emergency medical services (and later executive director of the West Virginia Pharmacists Association), phoned and instructed Steve to ground the helicopter. "It was late in the evening when the pilot walked in to pick up the medical supplies," Steve related. "When I told him he was grounded, he responded, 'Nobody grounds me, buddy,' turned around, carried the supplies to the helicopter and took off to fly the insulin to Petersburg... Every one of those helicopter pilots was a hero," Steve later said.

Marlinton wasn't the only West Virginia city hit by the 1985 flood. Franklin, Petersburg, and Rowlesburg also sustained extensive damage that November. The Petersburg/Moorefield area was hit by a severe flood caused by a rare hurricane that came up the valley and dropped fourteen inches of rain in 24 hours. Several deaths resulted, including Margaret Lilly Painter, a WVU School of Pharmacy alumnus of the class of 1979. Margaret and her husband were returning to their home in Elkins from Washington, D.C. where they had run in the Marine Corps Marathon. Caught by the rapidly rising water, they sought out a house on higher ground. After climbing onto the roof, Margaret was tragically swept away by the floodwater. Her husband, also swept away, managed to cling to a tree and was eventually saved. Margaret's body was recovered the following spring.[3]

Steve Judy, a pharmacist in Petersburg and owner of Judy's Pharmacy, recalled the flood as a "devastation that was unreal." When Steve arrived at his pharmacy during the flood to fill prescriptions, he found a number were for people other than his patients, such as Veterans Administration Hospital patients in Martinsburg who were traveling through the area at the time. Concerned about the limited supply of drugs he had available, Steve provided them with enough medication to get home. When the water receded, Steve found that both the bridge in Petersburg and the one between Moorefield and Petersburg had been destroyed. That afternoon, Air National Guard helicopters landed about 600 yards from his pharmacy and the Guard used an open space behind Steve's warehouse as a storage area for fuel and a service area for motor vehicles. Runners from the helicopters brought Steve prescription bottles from other pharmacies to be refilled, adding to his drug supply problem. A nearby Presbyterian church served as the food center for the area. For the next few days, Steve and his staff remained in the pharmacy and provided medical care to residents around the clock, taking turns sleeping wherever they could find a spot. When the water receded, Steve drove to his Moorefield pharmacy to assess the damage there. Finding minimal water damage at that pharmacy, he had it up and running in a few days. To supply medications to Steve's pharmacies, a wholesaler in Virginia had to route trucks through Maryland to Keyser, West Virginia. From there, Steve and his staff transported the parcels by automobile to Petersburg. The National

Guard delivered a tractor-trailer load of bottled water, cups, plates, and cleaning supplies that were distributed to residents from Steve's parking lot. Meanwhile, Steve's wife, a medical technologist at the local hospital, was one of many hospital employees who helped clean wounds and administer tetanus shots to limit infection. For the first five days after the flood, pharmacists and their staffs provided medical care to residents of the South Branch (Potomac River) Valley around the clock. According to Steve, "When it was all over, *Drug Topics* gave us an award 'for survival under less than perfect circumstances,' or something like that. It was an experience I shall never forget." [4]

Robert E. Proudfoot was born and reared in Rowlesburg, where his uncle had practiced medicine a generation earlier. Through high school, he worked in the local pharmacy performing such tasks as stoking the fire of the potbellied stove on early winter mornings and tending the soda fountain after school. Returning from overseas duty in the U.S. Army during World War II, Bob enrolled in the WVU School of Pharmacy and graduated in 1950. Following an internship with Dr. Roy Bird Cook in Charleston, Bob purchased a pharmacy in nearby Oakland, Maryland, where his practice thrived. Bob's son, Milton, also a registered pharmacist, had joined Bob prior to the November 1985 flood. [5]

At 8 PM on November 4, the Cheat River at Rowlesburg began to rise. By midnight, the water had overflowed its banks. [6] The 130-year old railroad trestle that spanned the river near the center of town was washed off its piers and fell into the riverbed. Storm debris collected in the bridge superstructure to form a funnel, diverting the water flow up Main Street like it was shot from the nozzle of a hose. Two blocks of the business district and two thirds of the houses in "the flats" (nearest the river bank) were damaged or destroyed by the water's impact. Residents of "the flats" escaped by climbing a hill overlooking the town where they were sheltered in homes of friends. [7]

Remembering with fondness the town where he lived as a youth, Bob Proudfoot returned to Rowlesburg and spent a month hosing down walls and providing whatever help he could for the people of the town. It was a sad homecoming for Bob. Long-time friends were now homeless and the house where he was born was destroyed. The residents of Rowlesburg hailed Bob as a hero. Although the disaster in Rowlesburg was bad, it still did not compare to the devastation experienced 40 years earlier in Shinnston. [5]

Charlie Stump was born in 1943 in Mullens, West Virginia, and graduated from the West Virginia University School of Pharmacy in the class of 1966. Charlie was a well-respected and popular pharmacist, his popularity a result of the services he provided to the community. He was also a modest man who did not seek recognition for his accomplishments. Without hesitation, Charlie would return to his pharmacy in Mullens after hours to fill prescriptions for a patient released late in the day from the hospital. It wasn't until after his untimely death following an automobile accident that his daughter, Eva (Stump) Burns, also a pharmacist and West Virginia University alumnus, became aware of the many facets of her father's community spirit. She learned her father who had long been involved with the youth of the county, once rented a bus to take the Mullens high school football team to a West Virginia University football game. She also discovered Charlie had anonymously deposited money into a customer's bank account so he could afford to get a prescription filled. In addition, Charlie paid the insurance premiums of several local residents after the devastating flood of 2001 to prevent their loss of coverage. [8]

The flood struck Mullens on July 8, 2001, and Charlie was both a victim and a hero. It rained so hard that day the main street of Mullens was converted into a river. Charlie's Pharmacy, owned by Charlie, was completely destroyed after being submerged under eight feet of muddy water.

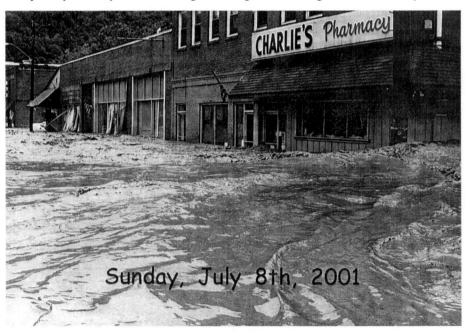

Charlie's Pharmacy

Eva Burns remembers: "The flood basically wiped out the whole downtown area. The damage was so extensive several buildings had to be torn down. Many others had to be gutted using sledgehammers in order to be rebuilt. A number of other homes were condemned." Charlie owned another pharmacy in nearby Pineville that fortunately escaped flood damage. Prescriptions were routed through Pineville until Charlie could acquire temporary space in Mullens for use as a pharmacy. Once the prescriptions were filled in Pineville, two of Charlie's pharmacy technicians brought them to Mullens and personally delivered them to the patients' homes. He then acquired a doublewide trailer that served as a temporary pharmacy. The damage in Mullens was so extensive Charlie was tempted to cut his losses and walk away, but such thoughts were short lived. Feeling the community had been good to him, Charlie felt he had an obligation to give back to the community. When he rebuilt, Charlie constructed a larger pharmacy designed to better serve his patients.[9]

Ethel Lusk was one of Charlie Stump's pharmacy technicians. She started working for Charlie in 1995 after completing her technician training at his pharmacy. "Although Charlie was a tough task maker, he was a good boss," Ethel recalled. "He was demanding, but if you did your work you got a pat on the back." Charlie Stump was always considerate of his employees. When Ethel's mother was dying of cancer, Charlie would suggest she "take an hour or so off to spend with her mother." Ethel adds, "When my dad was sick, I quit for six months to take care of him. Charlie would call and frequently come to the house to check on my dad. [Though] I quit my job in October, Charlie brought my Christmas bonus to my home in December." Ethel then told of the very old piano in the church that both she and Charlie attended. Charlie would tell Ethel, "We're going to get a new piano at the church one of these days." On one Saturday morning Charlie suggested to Ethel that she go over to the church and 'tell him what she thought.' Ethel asked Charlie what he expected her to see, to which he replied, 'Just go to the church and look around.' When she arrived, Ethel found that Charlie had bought a new piano for the church but didn't want the public to know who had given it. Ethel concluded, "He was a giant of a man."[10]

Charlie Stump died in February 2004. After his death, a pall fell over the community. According to Ethel, "some of his patients couldn't even come into the pharmacy because they just fell apart. They would call on the phone and cry. Mullens was absolutely devastated. It was unusual for one person to make the difference he did. There was such a showing of admiration and respect in the church at his wake. More than 1,500 people attended his funeral. Local citizens displayed ribbons on their doors in his remembrance. Charlie was buried at Hinton next to his mother. It was amazing how many people made that long trip to the cemetery at Hinton. Mullens had lost a hero."[9] Charlie was a rural pharmacist who truly touched the lives of the citizens in the community he loved and served.

Born in May 1954, Al Carolla is a 1980 graduate of the WVU School of Pharmacy, the fourth in his family to practice pharmacy. Al, who practices in southern McDowell county, recalls the floods of 2001 and 2002 from a different perspective. As a volunteer fireman and first responder, Al's story is told through the eyes of a fireman.[10] "The first flood occurred early one Sunday morning. Our area was nearly by-passed …we got only the edge of the storm. Suddenly all the pagers started going off at the fire department. Welch and Keystone, in the northern part of the county, were flooded. Each fire department was asked to respond as best it could. With that first flood, we played [only] a minor role by supplying water from our tanker trucks." The second flood, however, required much more from Al and his fellow firemen. It came in the spring of 2002 and resulted in about six inches of water in Al's pharmacy. After cleaning the store, Al went to the police department to assist the search and rescue efforts. Using four-wheel drive vehicles, Al and the others drove through the hollows trying to locate those people who had not been heard from. For the rest of that week, they went from house to house checking on the elderly since most of the roads were inaccessible. All three of the roads leading to Al's town were blocked with mountains of dirt and debris literally sitting in the middle of the highway. Large trees were stuck in the mud, blocking the roads and isolating the community. The State Road Commission was unable to reach the area to clear the roads for several days, so Al and the others along with coal miners used their mining equipment to open up the roads. Al assisted in supplying the people with needed medicine, drinking water and other supplies until conditions returned to normal.[10]

Al has been a volunteer fireman since 1989. When asked why he became a volunteer fireman, Al's response was unique. "It kinda' got thrown into my lap. I ran for mayor of Bradshaw one year against a man who was a consummate politician. My opponent's buddies were in the fire department, so when I won the election they all quit in protest. When I went over to check the equipment at the fire department, I saw I was not only mayor, but also the fire department! I have been here ever since." Apparently the other firemen were upset that Al, a Pennsylvanian who had only been in West

Virginia for about five years when the flood occurred, won the election for mayor. Although Al had wanted to be the mayor, after he was elected he was not enamored with the job. He became an emergency responder and fireman by default, but ultimately loved the challenge. When asked why he continued to serve as a volunteer fireman, Al's response was typical of a pharmacist: "There is no pay in it and it requires a lot of time and training. Hazmat training — training in handling hazardous materials -- takes a lot of time. In addition to floods, we get called for car wrecks and drug overdoses. The role of the fireman in each instance is that of a first responder. We stabilize the patient prior to transport. The satisfaction you derive from helping others makes the job worthwhile. Appreciation is shown when you help someone else. That's the pay you get." Today Al serves on the city council and has been with the fire department for 18 years. [10]

Arvel Wyatt is a pharmacist in Welch, West Virginia. Born in January 1937, he enlisted in the U.S. Air Force after graduating from high school. Assigned to a yearlong pharmacy course at Gunter Air Force Base in Montgomery, Alabama, Arvel spent the remainder of his four-year enlistment working in base hospital pharmacies in Japan. Enjoying his pharmacy experience in the service, he was accepted by the West Virginia University School of Pharmacy following discharge from the Air Force and received a Bachelor of Science degree in 1963. After graduation, he returned home to Welch where he joined Joe Monti and Buck Ireson in community pharmacy practice at the Flat Iron Drug Store. [11]

Reflecting back on the floods of 2001 and 2002, Arvel says, "Elkhorn Creek became congested with debris that caused it to overflow its banks and diverted [the flow of water] through the town. The water came shooting between buildings to the front door of our store. The force of the stream of water was so great it knocked the front door out, shot through the store and out the other side. Merchandise was floating in water, showcases were destroyed, and items from the store were later found a mile away." The area had two chain pharmacies, but Arvel's was the region's only independent pharmacy. The public's desire for an independent pharmacy prompted him to reopen rather than retire from practice. The chain stores refilled Arvel's patients' prescriptions while he was closed. Arvel had to buy new showcases, build new counters, and completely restock the pharmacy. Within three months, however, Arvel's pharmacy was reopened and ready for business, to the surprise of even the members of the West Virginia State Board of Pharmacy. Most, if not all, of Arvel's former patients returned, along with many new patients. In fact, some of Arvel's patients actually offered to help him rebuild and prepare the pharmacy for business.[11]

Then Governor Bob Wise visited Arvel on two occasions. After the first flood in 2001, the state awarded him a $20,000 grant that was forgivable provided Arvel remain in business for five or more years. Eight months later when the second flood destroyed Arvel's pharmacy, Governor Wise returned and mentioned the grant program. When Arvel pointed out the previous grant he received, Governor Wise forgave the first $20,000 on the spot and provided Arvel with a second $20,000 grant. In addition, Arvel received a small business loan at 1% interest. With the state's assistance and public support, Arvel was able to reopen his pharmacy and is busier than ever before.[11]

Each of these nine pharmacists shared a strong sense of community service accompanied by profound humility. West Virginia is proud of all of her pharmacist heroes.

Part Three

Shapers of Each Generation

Chapter Seven

Deans

Pharmacy education had a difficult beginning in West Virginia. In hindsight, one might wonder what possessed Joseph Lester Hayman, the first dean of the West Virginia University College of Pharmacy,[a] to accept the position when it was offered. Three prior attempts to develop a pharmacy program on the West Virginia University campus had failed. In 1899 and again in 1904, courses were offered in the University's catalog, but unfortunately no students applied. The third time, in 1914, Gordon A. Bergy was hired at the rank of instructor as the only other faculty member to teach in a newly created pharmacy department headed by Professor C. H. Rogers of the medical school. No designated space was allotted for the new department; its classrooms were scattered around the campus. Two years later, Professor Rogers left the University to accept a position at the University of Minnesota. Lonely Instructor Bergy was then called to active duty in the Army's Chemical Warfare Service in 1918. With Bergy's departure, the Department of Pharmacy closed for the duration of the war. Unfortunately, no record exists of the number of students enrolled or their disposition when Instructor Bergy was called to active duty.

However, as fate would have it, in February 1919, Mr. Bergy was furloughed to the ROTC unit at West Virginia University, allowing him to reestablish the Department of Pharmacy. That fall, J. Lester Hayman joined Mr. Bergy to once again create a faculty of two, located in the red brick School of Medicine building on the downtown campus. The pharmacy program curriculum was originally introduced by Instructor Bergy in 1915 and was two years in length, culminating in a Ph.G. degree (Table 1). In 1920, the Department of Pharmacy moved to the basement of Woodburn Hall and began its gradual transition and independence from the School of Medicine.

---

[a] *The West Virginia Board of Governors changed the name of the College of Pharmacy to the School of Pharmacy effective July 1, 1958.*

Table 1

Pharmacy Degree Programs offered by WVU

Degree Program	Minimum Length of Study	Year Initiation	Year Ended
Pharmaceutical Graduate (Ph.G.)	2 years	1915	1931
Pharmaceutical Chemist (Ph.C.)	3 years	1927	1935
Bachelor of Science (B.S.)	4 years	1917	1964
Bachelor of Science (B.S.)	5 years	1962	2000
Post-Baccalaureate Pharm.D.	2 years	1993	2000
Track-in Pharm.D.	6 years	1996	2001
Non-Traditional Pharm.D.	Variable	1998	2006
Entry-Level Pharm.D.	6 years	1998	Present

J. Lester Hayman graduated from the University of Michigan in 1919 with two degrees, a Pharmaceutical Chemist (Ph.C.) and a Bachelor of Science (B.S.) degree. At Michigan, he was an outstanding student and had been awarded the coveted Charles R. Eckler Prize in Microscopic Pharmacognosy. Following graduation, he had offers to join the pharmacy faculties of Valparaiso University, Western Reserve University and West Virginia University. Accepting the latter position, his teaching career began at the WVU Department of Pharmacy of the School of Medicine. The following year, he married Alice Bennett of Ohio and subsequently had two children, both of whom died tragically at early ages.[1]

Nineteen twenty-two proved to be a pivotal year for J. Lester Hayman: he was promoted to assistant professor and granted licensure by the West Virginia State Board of Pharmacy. In that era, West Virginia had a number of single-practitioner pharmacies whose owners had difficulty obtaining relief pharmacists for a much needed vacation. J. Lester Hayman filled this void by devoting his summers to travel around the state providing coverage for these owner-pharmacists. In this manner, he maintained his competency as a pharmacist, provided a much-needed service to the profession statewide, and promoted good will towards the fledgling Department of Pharmacy. In 1922, Hayman went back to Michigan for post-graduate study and received a Master of Science degree in 1925.[2] Returning to West Virginia University once again, he was promoted to associate professor in 1928 and advanced to professor of pharmacognosy in 1935. A year later, the University Board of Governors abolished the Department of Pharmacy and established a new College of Pharmacy. Named director of the College at its inception, Hayman took the reins as dean in 1938.[3]

Pharmacy prior to World War II was, without doubt, a male-dominated profession. However, J. Lester Hayman had the foresight to see that pharmacy was also a career ideally suited for women. As the United States headed into war with the resulting draft and voluntary military service, class sizes plummeted. Yet, enrollment of women was slow to increase. By 1943, total pharmacy student enrollment dropped to 16 (less than a third of the prewar enrollment) of whom seven were female.

Post-war enrollment in pharmacy peaked in 1947 at 127, several times the average prewar enrollment and 50% higher than the current enrollment. The influx of students coincided with the introduction of the "G.I. Bill" that promoted and financed education for veterans. This was a mixed blessing for Dean Hayman, now confronted with a massive influx of a different type of student: veterans ranging in age from 22 to 36 years, more mature than recent high school graduates, often married with children, some having acquired undergraduate degrees before the war. Robert G. Walsh, for example, currently of Westover, West Virginia, was a schoolteacher prior to entering the army. Having admired his hometown pharmacist as a youth, the G.I. Bill gave him an opportunity to study pharmacy. Many students like Walsh had served from two to four years in the armed forces and were highly disciplined combat veterans who wanted to get on with their lives with the shortest possible delay. Clyde Reed (see Chapter 5) had served in the 27th Infantry Division on Saipan fighting the Japanese, Herman F. Slaughter had flown 33 missions over Germany as a bombardier in B-17s, and William C. Bias had served on a light cruiser that shelled Tokyo Bay. The rank of those veterans enrolled in pharmacy at West Virginia University in 1947 ranged from private first class to lieutenant colonel. Recalling that Dean Hayman and his expanded, intrepid faculty of four were working out of the limited basement space of Woodburn Hall, one can only marvel at how so many could be educated by so few in such inadequate facilities.

J. Lester Hayman differed from his successor deans by projecting an image of both an academician and a clinician. Of particular note was his active participation in the state pharmacy association. After Lester's return from Michigan, he joined the West Virginia Pharmaceutical Association (WVPA) and was elected its secretary-treasurer in 1926, a post he held for 23 years. He served as WVPA president in 1959–1960, the only WVU dean to preside over this Association. In recognition of his service to the WVPA,

Lester was selected in 1947 to be the first recipient of the Dr. James Hartley Beal Award, the WVPA's highest honor.

Under his leadership, the Cook-Hayman Museum at the WVU School of Pharmacy was opened, and Lester shares with Dr. Roy Bird Cook the honor of its name.

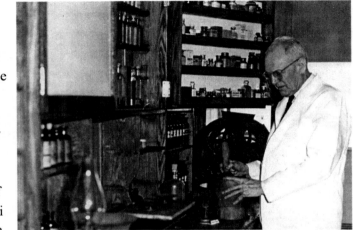

Dean J. Lester Hayman

Hayman retired from the School in July 1961 after 42 years of service to West Virginia, the University, and the pharmacy profession. Honored at the Annual School of Pharmacy Alumni Banquet that June, every pharmacist in the state was invited to attend, whether an alumnus or not. Close to 400 pharmacists accepted that invitation. Tragically, Professor J. Lester Hayman was involved in an automobile accident in Waterloo, Iowa, two years later and died July 6, 1963 from injuries sustained.[4]

Raphael Otto Bachmann succeeded Hayman as the second dean of the WVU School of Pharmacy and was the first dean of the School to hold a Ph.D. degree.[5] He assumed the responsibilities of professor and dean July 13, 1962. As dean, Bachmann was responsible for a number of firsts for the School. On arrival, Dean Bachmann discovered that the School lacked an on-going continuing education program that he deemed necessary for advancing pharmacy practice in the state. Thus, he and the faculty formed the "WVU Minutemen," so named because the faculty could develop a continuing education program on short notice at the request of county pharmacy societies. Twelve such programs were presented his first year. In conjunction with the WVPA, they also developed a two-day continuing education seminar presented each fall that was very popular with practicing pharmacists.[6]

By the third year of Dean Bachmann's tenure, faculty size grew to nine full time members. Although departments had yet to be formed, two faculty members taught pharmaceutics and another was hired to teach pharmacy practice and pharmacy administration coursework. The five-year curriculum was instituted in 1965 with 38 first year students enrolled,[7] an increase of three from the previous year. The five year program had concerned many practicing pharmacists throughout the state who feared that better students would shun pharmacy as a career should the curriculum be extended an extra year. Although the increased enrollment was modest, it was sufficient to alleviate the practitioners' anxiety.

The pharmacy school could afford to increase the number of entering freshmen through federal grants awarded based on first year enrollments. The newly implemented federal capitation program, called the Area Health Education Consortium (AHEC), applied to both schools of pharmacy and medicine and extended over a period of fifteen years.[8] During the years of University participation, AHEC generated over four million dollars that were applied to the development of the newly constructed Health Sciences Center.[9]

Ray Bachmann was a master at obtaining external funding for the School. During his tenure, the Gordon A. Bergy Lecture Series was initiated and sustained by utilizing alumni contributions. This lecture series features renowned pharmacy educators and scholars and continues to be supported by an endowment created by the Bergy family. Dr. Bachmann instituted a visiting scientist program that brought two nationally prominent lecturers to campus each year; however, this program no longer exists. A National Science Foundation grant was obtained to support a summer session and an undergraduate research program. A Fentom research grant to study tablet formulations was obtained, and faculty had fellowships supported by National Institutes of Health grants.[10] Under Dean Bachmann's leadership, a new era in research emerged to expand the horizons of the School.

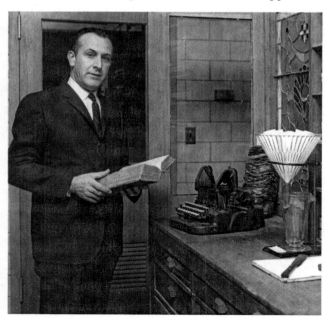

Dean Bachmann in Pharmacy Museum

A new Master of Science in Pharmacy degree program initiated under Dean Bachmann awarded its first degree in December 1968. By the fall of 1971, faculty size had grown to 18 and 61 students graduated that academic year from the Bachelor of Science degree program. Undergraduates began to take advantage of a broad spectrum of educational opportunities. Of the 61 graduates in 1972, 47 entered community pharmacy, 11 became hospital pharmacists, and three enrolled in the Master of Science graduate program, increasing the total enrollment in this program to six. With the assistance of a regional medical program grant, in 1972 the Drug Information Center was founded to provide drug information to health care professionals throughout the state and its first full time director, Dr. Arthur Jacknowitz, was recruited. The Center, under the name of the West Virginia Center for Drug and Health Information, continues to date with Dr. Marie Abate (see Chapter 12) as director. The School of Pharmacy under Dean Bachmann's insightful watch began to attract national recognition.

Things were to take a tragic turn for Dean Bachmann, however. At 51 years of age, he met an untimely death on December 18, 1972, due to a ruptured aortic aneurysm. Ray had provided visionary leadership to the School of Pharmacy throughout a period of major curricular change and rapid growth. He was a popular dean, and with his loss a sense of sadness descended over the institution. Dr. Frank O'Connell took over the reins as acting dean. A year later, on December 7, 1973, leadership was handed to Louis Anthony Luzzi, Ph.D., a Rhode Island native.

On becoming the third dean of the WVU School of Pharmacy, Dr. Luzzi had a plan to revise and expand the professional program and the fledgling graduate program. In his seven prior years as professor at the University of Georgia, Dr. Luzzi acquired a national reputation in pharmaceutics and served as a research consultant to several segments of the pharmaceutical industry. While at Georgia, he developed the U.S. Food and Drug Administration Inspector Training Course, a unique program designed solely to train newly hired FDA employees.[10] As a scientist, Dr. Luzzi recognized that a major deficit of the WVU School of Pharmacy was a lack of research publications and funding. However, Lou Luzzi had to contend with multiple forces pulling in several different directions. The State legislature insisted that a Charleston Division be established, the School lacked a Ph.D. program, and Dr. Luzzi perceived a need for a major administrative reorganization.

Starting with the latter, Dr. Luzzi organized an Academic Standards Committee, a Faculty Personnel Evaluation Committee, an Admissions

Committee, and a Curriculum Committee to evaluate educational needs. He established an Executive Committee consisting of the newly appointed associate dean, and the three academic specialty coordinators from the Clinical Sciences, Basic Pharmaceutical Sciences, and the Social and

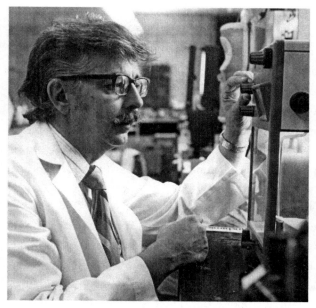

Managerial Sciences areas. A Charleston Division was ultimately established in 1977 with three clinical pharmacy faculty assigned to teach, provide patient care consultations, and operate a pharmacokinetics laboratory. The Bachelor of Science degree curriculum was revised with greater emphasis placed on clinical clerkships in a variety of practice

Dean Luzzi in Laboratory

areas.[11] During his deanship, faculty size further increased and student enrollment escalated because the previously mentioned federal capatation program provided subsidies based upon class size.

Dean Luzzi was well known and respected for his energy and enthusiasm, interest in developing new programs, and ability to mentor young faculty. A Ph.D. program was initiated in 1978 with the first Ph.D. awarded in 1982 in medicinal chemistry. Outreach activities, coordinated through the Drug Information Center, included tele-lectures as well as correspondence courses, and personal visitations were begun. Adjunct faculty and preceptors were appointed. Additionally, at the request of the State legislature, Dr. Luzzi initiated a program for the statewide purchasing of pharmaceutical items that allowed generic bidding while maintaining a high standard of quality. Over the first four years of this School-managed program, the unit drug cost generally decreased while the quality of drugs purchased improved. The program was considered to be a success.[12] Dr. Luzzi's leadership and willingness to experiment led the School of Pharmacy on a path to national recognition.[13]

With the construction of the Health Sciences Center in the late 1950s, a model pharmacy for teaching purposes had been built in conjunction with the School of Pharmacy. As WVU Hospital neared completion a few years later, the pharmacy school considered its options of either closing its pharmacy or keeping it open to serve outpatients at the Medical Center Clinics. Dr. Michael Musulin from the School of Pharmacy was asked by Dr. Luzzi to consult with local pharmacists to determine if any objected to a School-operated pharmacy at the Health Sciences Center. Since the outpatient pharmacy had been started with contributions from local pharmacists and the WVPA, Dr. Luzzi felt obligated to seek the approval of the community pharmacists.[14]

Prior to the opening of WVU Hospital in 1960, the School's outpatient pharmacy on the downtown campus could be described as a "shoebox operation" in that it was quite small and lacked any degree of sophistication. After WVU Hospital opened, the pharmacist in charge, Mrs. Clara Skarzinski, was relocated to the Medical Center campus and Mr. Douglas Gill took over the outpatient pharmacy and the downtown Student Health Service pharmacy, also under control of the hospital.[14] In time, the hospital ran into problems operating the outpatient pharmacy and wanted to divest itself of it. In 1979, Dr. Luzzi directed Drs. Bruce Berger and John Baldwin to evaluate the outpatient pharmacy operation. Their findings confirmed that the pharmacy was operating in the red and had been doing so for some time. What had saved the outpatient pharmacy was the coverage of its losses at the end of the year by the associate vice president for finance. A lack of attention to detail rather than malfeasance appeared to explain the loss, and the problem was soon corrected. However, the School of Pharmacy operation of the outpatient pharmacy would later become a tempest that escalated to storm proportions after Dr. Luzzi left the School.

Dr. Luzzi's initial concern about the School's weakness in research continued, despite the fact that as Dr. John Baldwin recalls, "…Dr. Luzzi had [already] taken …steps to put the School of Pharmacy on the map." [14] At that time, Dr. William Higuchi, an internationally recognized scientist, had an established research program at the University of Michigan that was well funded with federal grants. Dr. Higuchi had contacted Dr. Luzzi regarding the possibility of relocating to Morgantown along with his research staff. His reason for wanting to leave Michigan at that time was an existing space problem at the University of Michigan College of Pharmacy that was detrimental to his research. If recruited, Dr. Higuchi and his scientific reputation would undoubtedly lend prestige to West Virginia University. Not only was his program well funded but the grant money was transferable. If Dr. Higuchi came to WVU, the School of Pharmacy would acquire a fully funded, full time research scientist capable of addressing a major research deficit. To Dean Luzzi, this was an easy decision — Dr. Higuchi wanted to come to Morgantown and Dr. Luzzi was eager to have him. The Executive Committee was consulted and its members likewise agreed. Nonetheless, Dr. Charles Andrews, then vice president for health sciences at WVU, refused to provide space for Dr. Higuchi despite the obvious short and potentially long term advantages.[14] Little consideration was given to the School's gain of a full time research scientist/professor, a research staff, and a premier research program at little cost to the University. Dr. Andrews' stated reason for refusing the space request was based on salary considerations. The proposed salary for Dr. Higuchi would exceed that of Dean Luzzi, which Dr. Andrews considered to be improper even though Dr. Luzzi rejected this as inconsequential.[15] Dr. Higuchi was not hired, and he later accepted a position at the University of Utah College of Pharmacy.

The Higuchi matter made it clear to Dr. Luzzi that the School of Pharmacy lacked support from the Health Sciences Center's central administration, and he could not expect change in the foreseeable future. With this in mind, Dr. Luzzi made the decision to leave West Virginia University. Many faculty members were stunned when they learned of his plans. After a six-year tenure, he resigned his position at West Virginia University in June 1980 to accept an appointment as dean of the School of Pharmacy and provost for health sciences at his alma mater, the University of Rhode Island.[16] Again, Dr. Frank O'Connell stepped in to serve in the interim. After a long illness, Dean Luzzi died on May 12, 2007.

Sidney Alan Rosenbluth arrived in Morgantown as the fourth dean of the School of Pharmacy on August 1, 1981, a year following Dr. Luzzi's resignation. A native of Texas and professionally educated in Texas and Oklahoma, he had a unique doctoral background in pharmaceutics and biochemistry, extensive experience in the area of psychiatric pharmacy, a Master of Science degree in hospital pharmacy and a postdoctoral research fellowship in 1966 from Bath University in England.[17]

Dr. Rosenbluth was a faculty member at the University of Tennessee at Memphis, rising from assistant professor of pharmaceutics to professor of pharmaceutics and director of pharmacy affairs. He was director of pharmacy affairs at three hospitals: City of Memphis Hospital, the Tennessee Psychiatric Hospital and Institute, and the West Tennessee Chest Disease

Hospital.[17] With an interest in pharmaceutical research, Dr. Rosenbluth changed his professional and academic direction during his tenure at the University of Tennessee. He became a strong advocate for greater

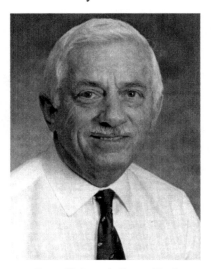

Dean Sidney A. Rosenbluth

pharmacist participation in the clinical well being of the patient with regard to both disease treatment and prevention. Recognizing the pharmacist's potential for input into clinical decision-making, Dr. Rosenbluth along with students initiated pharmacist interactions in outreach psychiatric facilities within the Memphis area.[18] In 1973, he became assistant dean for clinical affairs and later associate dean for student affairs before accepting the position of dean at WVU.

By the early 1980s, state-run university affiliated hospitals around the country were having financial problems. To address this issue, Mr. David Fine, West Virginia University hospital administrator, and vice president for health sciences Dr. Charles Andrews, formed a corporation in the early to mid 1980s. Mr. Fine, nationally recognized as a rising star in his field, developed a plan to dissociate the hospital from the University by forming a separate corporation. This was done with the support of the University president. Mr. Fine spent several months in Charleston lobbying for the divestiture bill. Dean Rosenbluth was asked by the hospital administrator to support this bill and to write a letter showing support by saying it would benefit the University. It wasn't until after the bill passed that Dean Rosenbluth had the opportunity to view the bill and realize he had been deceived.[19] The bill clearly stipulated that any moneymaking proposition associated with the Health Sciences Center would fall under the corporate domain, effective July 1, 1985.

Excess revenue after expenses from the outpatient pharmacy had been returned to the School prior to the divestiture. These monies provided graduate pharmacy student stipends, funded faculty and student travel expenses to meetings, and helped with laboratory equipment needs as well as other research efforts. The Drug Information Center had also been partially funded by excess revenue from the outpatient pharmacy, with the money helping to support a role-model learning environment for senior pharmacy students and the provision of information for multiple operations in the School of Pharmacy. Thus, the outpatient pharmacy had significantly contributed to the financial support of the School. A revenue budget of less than $200,000 in 1980 had grown to approximately $800,000 in 1985 due to improvements in net income, inventory, teaching loads of the pharmacy faculty and staff, patient services and efficiency.[19] With passage of the divestiture bill, all pharmacy revenue income reverted to the corporation. To the hospital administrators, control over the outpatient pharmacy was viewed as a "cash cow." Once the corporation gained control over the outpatient pharmacy, all functions not generating income were eliminated. Employees of the outpatient pharmacy felt betrayed and unappreciated, and many left.

As if the loss of a significant part of the School's financial support was not enough of a burden, Dr. Rosenbluth's administration was soon to be plagued by a major scandal: embezzlement by the School's office manager. In February 1992, a local newspaper article reported employee theft through a sophisticated scheme involving forgery, deposits to an employee controlled personal bank account, faked endorsements, and other forms of deceit in order to misappropriate funds. Over time, an investigation revealed that most of the dollars lost were WVU Foundation funds, not covered by the State's insurance. As a result of this experience, the University and State subsequently revised their financial controls and systems to ensure proper accountability. Unfortunately, the negative impact of the embezzlement significantly impacted alumni giving to the School, which required a number of years to overcome after Dr. Rosenbluth stepped down as dean.

Looking at the accomplishments of Dr. Rosenbluth during his tenure as dean from 1981 to 1994, he strongly believed in a greater role for the pharmacist in preventive and therapeutic disease management. He always applauded the successes of his students and staff. During his term as dean, tenure track faculty positions increased with an increase in the annual budget; departmental chairs were appointed to replace area coordinators; the School's Visiting Committee tripled in size to include representatives from industry and various professional practice pharmacists; the undergraduate research seminar, which drew undergraduate students from numerous states to present their research findings, became a national model for increasing student interest in research and graduate education; volunteer faculty affiliations, both preceptors and practice sites, more than doubled; the West Virginia Poison Center was certified as a regional center; the Ph.D. program was fully accepted as a University graduate degree in 1984; a Ph.D. program in Behavioral and Administrative Pharmacy was established; and Health

Sciences Center receipt of a Kellogg award allowed the School of Pharmacy to place faculty and provide services at multiple rural health sites. With subsequent support from the Caperton plan (from then Governor Gaston Caperton), undergraduate students were able to gain experiences in these rural practice sites.

Dr. Rosenbluth stepped down as dean in 1994 to accept an appointment as AACPs Scholar in Residence for 1994–1995. After completion of this appointment, Dr. Rosenbluth returned to the University as professor. He retired from the School's faculty on August 31, 2001, as professor emeritus.

George Robert Spratto, Ph.D., arrived in Morgantown as the fifth dean of the West Virginia University School of Pharmacy on June 29, 1995. Dr. Spratto received a Bachelor of Science in pharmacy degree from Fordham University in 1961 and a Ph.D. in pharmacology at the University of Minnesota in 1966. After graduation from the University of Minnesota, Dr. Spratto accepted a position with the Food and Drug Administration (FDA) in the Bureau of Drug Abuse Control and the Bureau of Narcotics and Dangerous Drugs for two years.[20]

Upon leaving the FDA, Dr. Spratto entered academia as an assistant professor at Purdue University in 1968. Over the next 27 years, he advanced to professor and subsequently served as associate dean for professional programs at Purdue University School of Pharmacy and Pharmacal Sciences. Since opportunity for further advancement at Purdue was uncertain, he accepted an invitation to visit West Virginia University and interviewed for the position of dean.[20] Although he was fully aware of a number of existing problems at the WVU School of Pharmacy, Dr. Spratto believed they could be overcome and welcomed the challenge.[21]

After arriving as dean, Dr. Spratto embarked upon an 18-month plan for his administration that included: improving communications and cooperation among faculty (which had become a growing problem); addressing the individual goals of faculty members; developing and implementing an entry-level Pharm.D. program; hiring a chair of the Department of Basic Pharmaceutical Sciences (at that time filled by an interim chair); enhancing declining alumni relations which had become critical due to the embezzlement; improving inadequate teaching laboratory facilities and upgrading research laboratories; and establishing a strategic plan (none existed at that time).

Dr. Spratto's first consideration was to develop a Pharm.D. curriculum that met the needs of the students and ultimately West Virginia and the profession. This was achieved under his administration, and plans to continually enhance the curriculum are ongoing. Alumni relations markedly improved under Dean Spratto's guidance, with the attainment by the School of a previously unprecedented level of donor support and external funding. Significant renovation of the physical plant was accomplished. Of particular note, funds were received to construct a state of the art Center for Pharmaceutical Care Education funded by Mylan Laboratories, which greatly improved teaching and laboratory capabilities. Other achievements have resulted in increased office space and improved research laboratories. The graduate program also significantly improved and expanded.

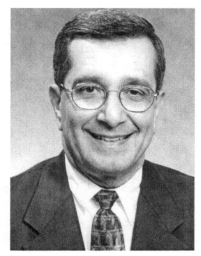

Dean George Spratto

In 2003, Dean Spratto assisted in the creation of a new school of pharmacy in conjunction with the Oman Medical College in Muscat, Oman. Most of his efforts were in curriculum development and faculty hiring. Cooperation with the Oman Medical College was part of an undertaking by the West Virginia University Health Sciences Center to advance modern medicine and health care in a developing Middle Eastern country. Dr. Spratto had previously been a member of a U.S. evaluation team working with the Ministry of Health, United Arab Emirates, to review the pharmacy programs at Ajman University's three campuses (Ajman, Al Ain, and Abu Dhabi) for accreditation by their Ministry of Health.

Despite his many accomplishments, Dr. Spratto experienced some disappointments at West Virginia University.[21] Foremost was an inability to significantly increase faculty salaries. "Salaries," he stated, "are increasing yearly at the national level, but not at WVU. We do not keep up with the national average. Whereas at other institutions the faculty may receive a 5-7% raise, here raises are closer to 2%." Another need was significant funding for research as well as for renovating more research laboratories. Even with the significant external funding obtained, a larger percentage of alumni still needed to contribute in order to allow for continual, ongoing enhancement of School programs. Nonetheless, the School was in much better shape upon his departure as dean compared to its state when he arrived.

Upon his retirement to Connecticut in summer 2006, Dr. Spratto became a professor emeritus with the WVU School of Pharmacy and continues to write and edit the <u>Nurse's Drug Handbook</u> as he has for the past 30 years. Dr. Spratto also continues to serve his appointment as a member of the

Accreditation Council for Pharmacy Education (ACPE) and he assumed the role as ACPE president for 2007-2008.

In the 70 years since the West Virginia University College of Pharmacy was established and the more than 85 years of pharmaceutical education in West Virginia, five deans have served with devotion and distinction. Each of these men made major contributions to pharmacy education in the State. J. Lester Hayman provided the organizational leadership for the fledgling school. He led it through two major transformation periods in the pharmacy profession, from the compounding and herbal remedy dominance that characterized pre-World War II, through the era of rapid and immoderate change post-World War II. Raphael O. Bachmann provided leadership for the School in its early years of faculty and student proliferation as well as curricular change that was responsible for new initiatives such as the Drug Information Center, the Master of Science program, and graduate research. Louis A. Luzzi led the School through its maturation years by fostering campus expansion, delineating departments, and developing clinical clerkships. He initiated a new Ph.D. program in 1978 that was officially recognized by the University during the succeeding dean's tenure. Sidney A. Rosenbluth advocated a greater role for the pharmacist in disease prevention and management and initiated another Ph.D. program. George R. Spratto

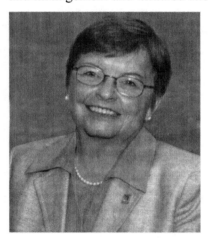

Dean Patricia Chase

brought stability to the fragmented School that existed upon his arrival and raised the School to a new level of alumni support and external funding. He was also responsible for significant infrastructure enhancements that improved teaching and research. Dean Patricia Chase was appointed July 1, 2006, as the first female dean of the School. Her task will be to continue the program of excellence that her predecessors developed and nurtured. It is anticipated that her tenure will continue the productivity and innovation of her predecessors.

In the years ahead, the WVU School of Pharmacy will likely face new and unforeseen challenges in the face of rapid and continuing technological advances and increasingly fragile national and global environments. With these challenges, however, will also come unprecedented opportunities. The echoes of the past need to be heard by the future leaders of the School so its proud legacy will continue.

Chapter Eight

Emeritus Faculty

Webster's New International Dictionary defines the term "emeritus" as "holding after retirement (as from professional or academic office) an honorary title corresponding to that held last during active service, especially after gaining public or professional recognition, a...college professor." [1] The School of Pharmacy of West Virginia University has been blessed through the years with a premier faculty, several of whom provided many years of loyal service. However, many of their records are "bare bones," consisting solely of lists of accomplishments devoid of commentary. The University introduced the title "Emeritus" in the decade of the 1970s, although the exact year is unknown. Since that time, two deans and five faculty members have been granted official emeritus status. One additional dean and two professors fulfill the Webster definition, although the service of two of these individuals preceded the 1970s. Considering all of these faculty and deans provided many years of exemplary service to the University, their stories deserve to be told.

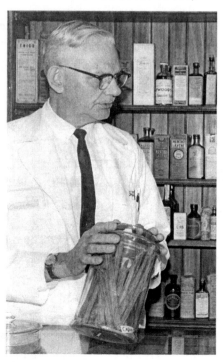

Professor Geiler in Pharmacy Museum

Frederick Linck Geiler was the first WVU School of Pharmacy faculty member to be honored with emeritus status. The first notice of this appointment was found in the West Virginia University Bulletin in April 1974, three years after he retired from WVU. Fred was born on November

5, 1901, in Portsmouth, Scio County, Ohio. As an undergraduate at The Ohio State University, he was active in the Army ROTC. The 1928 Ohio State yearbook, *The Makio,* lists Fred as President Brigade Colonel 4 (presumably cadet colonel) as well as a member of the Pershing Rifles, Scabbard and Blade, and the Cadet Officers Club. Following his graduation with a Bachelor of Science degree in 1928, Fred joined the faculty of the Department of Pharmacy of the West Virginia University School of Medicine as the Department's third member, with the rank of instructor. In 1930, his third year on the faculty, Fred was elected to membership in the Tau Chapter of Phi Lambda Upsilon Honorary Chemical Society. That same year, he married Beatrice Margaret Babb, two years his elder. When the Department of Pharmacy was re-established in 1936 as the College of Pharmacy, the faculty size had not changed from the preceding eight years. Fred taught pharmaceutical dispensing with ancillary duties of editing the *Showglobe,* a publication for pharmacy alumni. In June 1935, Fred received a Master of Science degree from West Virginia University and was promoted to assistant professor in 1937. Geiler achieved the rank of associate professor in 1944 and was further promoted to professor in 1951.

Fred was an imposing figure standing well over six feet tall, with a full head of graying hair and a neatly trimmed mustache. He was usually positioned in the center of the back row in group photographs. Fred has been described as the quintessential "German Professor," demanding and formal.[2] He walked with a limp but no one knew why. Although his voice was not loud, it was penetrating. He was meticulous in everything he did and impressed upon his students to follow his example. One day Fred confronted a student who had been unable to answer a question in his class all week. Fred asked the student how he could expect to get through pharmacy school with so little knowledge, to which the student replied, "Pharmacy school? I'm supposed to be in forestry school." He then arose, took his books and left the classroom.[3]

In his dispensing laboratory, Fred emphasized the filling of prescriptions with precision and neatness. The typed label must be free from strikeovers and affixed to the bottle so it was centered and absolutely straight. Woe to the student whose prescription bottle bore a smudge or fingerprint! Alcohol was always doled out to the precise milliliter. There was a day the class was making Lemon Peel Tincture. It was hot and humid and Professor Geiler announced to the class they could make lemonade with any left over lemons. Unbeknownst to Geiler, as the lemonade production progressed, everyone's grain alcohol mysteriously "evaporated." Professor Geiler, noticing the happy students but none the wiser, commented that a little lemonade could certainly improve a student's mood.[4]

Professor Geiler was known for his matter-of-fact sense of humor. Tom Traubert, a former student, tells how one day in Fred's laboratory he failed to close a bottom lab desk drawer. Tom was busy and didn't see Professor Geiler approaching his desk. Failing to notice the open drawer, Professor Geiler hit his shin on the drawer as he walked by. Although nothing was said at the time, Fred's facial expression indicated he was in great pain. Five years later as an alumnus, Tom visited the School. When Professor Geiler saw Tom he reminded him of the event and, with a twinkle in his eye, added that his leg still bothered him after all that time. On another occasion, Tom was sitting in class tilting back his chair when the chair fell over. Professor Geiler remarked, "Traubert, I don't mind if you go to sleep in my class but try not to disturb the rest of us." [5]

In 1960, Fred was made an honorary alumnus of West Virginia University School of Pharmacy, which speaks for itself in that the University does not routinely make such appointments. He was awarded the Outstanding Service Award in 1966 and retired in 1971 after 43 years of service to the School. During that year, he also received the Dr. James H. Beal Award, the West Virginia Pharmacists Association's highest honor. On retirement, Fred moved to Napoleon, Michigan, where he died May 22, 1979.

Sixteen years elapsed between Fred Geiler's appointment as the first emeritus professor of pharmacy and Frank O'Connell's appointment as the second. Frank Dennis O'Connell was born in Lynn, Massachusetts, in July 1927. Following graduation from high school, Frank entered the U.S. Army as an enlisted man, serving in the Army of Occupation in Berlin, Germany, from January to December 1946. Enrolling in the bachelor of science in pharmacy degree program at Massachusetts College of Pharmacy in 1947, he graduated in 1951 and earned a Master of Science degree in pharmaceutical chemistry from that institution in 1953. Frank was elected to membership in the Rho Chi Honor

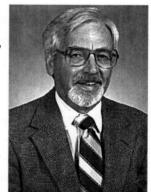

Professor Frank O'Connell

Society as an undergraduate and to the Sigma Xi Honor Society as a graduate student. Frank served as a research foundation fellow at Purdue University from 1956 to 1957, earning a Ph.D. in pharmacognosy in 1957.

A fellow graduate student in Indiana recruited Frank for West Virginia University. Frank was told WVU was building a new medical center and he should look into job possibilities there. He recalls arriving in Morgantown in 1957 for the job interview, finding the medical center was still under construction and the University Hospital was represented by a crater in the ground. For his first year and a half, Frank taught in Science (now Martin) Hall at Woodburn Circle on the main campus. Initially he was given the "odds and ends" courses to teach, such as pharmaceutical calculations, and as a junior faculty member he helped out with other courses. After Frank organized his pharmacognosy course, his faculty designation was changed from assistant professor of pharmacy to assistant professor of pharmacognosy. Six years later at the recommendation of Dean Bachmann, he was promoted to associate professor of pharmacognosy. Frank then achieved the rank of professor of pharmacognosy in 1968. Following the untimely death of Dean Bachmann in the fall of 1972, he was appointed acting dean for the first time, a position he held until Dr. Louis Luzzi was hired as dean. The following year, Frank was honored by the American Society of Pharmacognosy by being elected their national treasurer. When Louis A. Luzzi arrived, he recommended Frank for the positions of assistant dean and director of the drug abuse program at West Virginia University. Frank also served on the task force to rewrite the state pharmacy law. Frank was called upon a second time to serve as acting dean when Dr. Luzzi left WVU for Rhode Island in 1980, prior to Alan Rosenbluth's arrival as dean. Once again, Frank worked to maintain the operation of the School during this transition period. Frank was promoted to associate dean under Dean Rosenbluth, a position he maintained until his retirement. By 1986, Frank's courses in chemotherapeutic and immunobiologic agents and radiopharmacy, along with his lecture on AIDS therapy, had become key components of the didactic curriculum, unfortunately to the exclusion of the teaching of pharmacognosy. But, changing times had relegated pharmacognosy to the "dust bin of history," somewhat ironic given the widespread use of natural products today. Frank accepted the inevitable and gave up hope of restoring a course on pharmacognosy and herbal medicine in the curriculum.[6] Today this information is interspersed throughout the curriculum.

Frank O'Connell retired from full time teaching on June 30, 1990. He was granted the title of professor emeritus effective July 1, 1990, in recognition of his many contributions to the School of Pharmacy during his 33 years of service. In particular, Frank was the first member of the pharmacy faculty to be granted a sabbatical leave, during which he enrolled at the University of Southern California to obtain experience in dispensing dosage forms for nuclear medicine. After Frank retired, six years elapsed before Dr. David Riley became the third faculty member to receive emeritus status.

David Allen Riley is a West Virginia native, born in Bridgeport on May 4, 1938. Dr. Riley enrolled in the West Virginia University School of Pharmacy in 1956 and received a Bachelor of Science degree in pharmacy and a commission as Second Lieutenant in the U.S. Air Force Reserve in 1961. David worked as a staff pharmacist in Uniontown, Pennsylvania, for a year until ordered to report for a three-year tour of active duty as chief pharmacy officer, medical squadron commander, and hospital registrar at the Amarillo Air Force Base in Texas. David worked as a manufacturers' representative for a year after completing his service obligation followed by nine years in community pharmacy practice in Texas, Georgia, and West Virginia. However, having tired

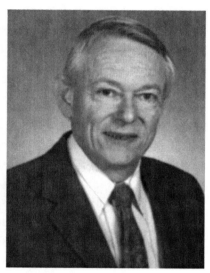

Professor David Riley

feet was not to David's liking, leading to the realization that community pharmacy was not the profession for him. In 1971, David earned a Master of Science degree in pharmacy administration and entered academic pharmacy at the University of Georgia as coordinator of continuing education programs in pharmacy, an area that would remain his focus for the rest of his career. A doctorate in education followed in 1975, at which time David followed his mentor, Dr. Lou Luzzi, to West Virginia to take a position as interim chair of the Department of Behavioral and Administrative Pharmacy at West Virginia University until a permanent chair could be hired.

As director of continuing education at the WVU School of Pharmacy, David organized 32 continuing education programs during his 20 years of University service. He honored two of his professors, Drs. Albert Wojcik and Frank O'Connell, with an annual alumni seminar dedicated to their teaching and research areas. He also planned and organized symposia given throughout the state and at distant locations. David tells of one such program, the First International Symposium on Microencapsulation, that was held in

Miami, Florida. Typical of Murphy's Law, the week before the symposium was scheduled the hotel burned. David hurriedly arranged for another hotel, but time was insufficient to notify attendees from Europe, Canada, and Japan. Improvising as best he could, David stood at the airport with a sign to notify the registrants of the hotel change as they arrived for the symposium.

The WVU School of Pharmacy honored David by selecting him as its 1979 Outstanding Alumnus. On retirement, he received a Certificate of Appreciation from Governor Gaston Caperton for 25 years of loyal and dedicated service to West Virginia. His dedication to education has remained to the present time. Twenty-nine years ago David helped his long time friend, Harvey Whitney, publisher of the *Annals of Pharmacotherapy* and the *Journal of Pharmacy Technology,* develop criteria for the certification of articles for continuing education accreditation by the American Association of Colleges of Pharmacy. He chaired the Continuing Education Committee for 28 years before retiring from reviewing manuscripts and organizing activities. David retired on August 1, 1996, receiving emeritus professor status on retirement.[7] The following year he received the William L. Blockstein Award of Merit, presented by the Eli Lilly Company on behalf of the Continuing Education Section of the American Association of Colleges of Pharmacy. He currently resides in Morgantown with his wife, Janet. A year following David Riley's retirement, Dr. James K. Lim was named the fourth professor emeritus.

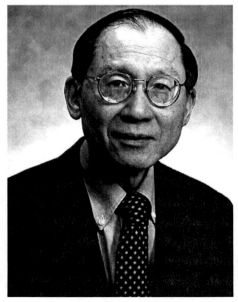
Professor James Lim

Born in Indonesia, James K. Lim received his early education in Singapore, earning a Bachelor of Pharmacy degree from the University of Malaya (now Malaysia) in 1953. Emigrating to the United States, he enrolled at the University of North Carolina where he earned a Master of Science degree in pharmaceutics in 1962 and a Ph.D. in 1965. Dr. Lim's teaching career began at West Virginia University with an appointment as assistant professor of pharmaceutics in July 1966. Thirty-one years later he retired as emeritus professor having served as the interim chair of the Department of Basic Pharmaceutical Sciences and interim coordinator of the graduate program. Jim, usually referred to as Jimmy by many of his faculty colleagues, was known for his kind and gentle manner, his always warm and friendly greetings, and his ever smiling demeanor.

During his professional career, Jim taught nine undergraduate and five graduate courses covering the areas of pharmaceutics, cosmetic formulation, manufacturing, and nutrition. He mentored 17 Master of Science degree candidates, three Ph.D. candidates and three post-doctoral research fellows. He conducted research work in semisolid rheology, sustained release formulations, and dental plaque anti-adherents. Jim served as Secretary of the University Faculty Senate and chair of the Welfare Committee. He is credited for the formation of the Faculty Mediation Program at WVU.

Reflecting back on his years in academia, Dr. Lim's most precious moments were his interactions with students. "We no longer emphasize the basics to the students, as we did in the past," he laments. "As time elapsed classes grew larger, and the close personal relationships between faculty and students diminished noticeably. I believe, in a way, we lost the flavor of traditional pharmacy. Students show their appreciation to their mentors in different ways, but the respect of a student is the greatest reward a teacher can receive." Dr. James K. Lim retired as emeritus professor of pharmaceutics on July 1, 1997, with the respect of his students and fellow faculty. He currently lives in Great Falls, Virginia.[8]

Carl Joseph Malanga, the next emeritus faculty member, was born August 26, 1939, in New York City. After enrolling at Fordham University College of Pharmacy, he excelled as a student, graduating *Magna Cum Laude* with a Bachelor of Science degree in pharmacy in 1961 and as a Distinguished Military Graduate that entitled him to a regular army commission as a Second Lieutenant. As an undergraduate, Carl received the Borden Outstanding Freshman Prize, the Merck Award and the Bristol

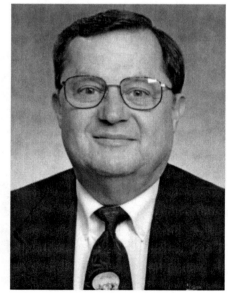

Professor Carl Malanga

Award, was elected to Rho Chi Honor Society and was chosen valedictorian of the class of 1961. From 1962 to 1964, Carl served in the U.S. Army as a company grade infantry officer, rising to the rank of First Lieutenant. For the next three years after completing his service obligation (he had declined a regular army commission), Carl enrolled in the Department of Biological Sciences graduate school at Fordham University while he served in the active reserve as a training officer in the Medical Service Corps. He received a Master of Science degree in 1967 followed by a Ph.D. in 1970.

Early in his last semester at Fordham University, Carl arranged a job interview at West Virginia University with Dean Ray Bachmann. He flew from New York to Pittsburgh in terrible weather and took a commuter flight from Pittsburgh after a long delay due to fog. After several aborted attempts to land in Morgantown, the pilot flew to Clarksburg but the ceiling was too low, causing them to return to Pittsburgh. On that flight, Carl had a conversation with a fellow passenger who inquired about the nature of his business in Morgantown. Interestingly, that passenger was Gene Staples, the C.E.O. of the West Virginia University Hospital. Upon hearing Carl was to interview at the School of Pharmacy, Staples suggested they travel together. As the airline attempted to arrange ground transportation, a cardiologist from the School of Medicine whose wife had just departed on an overseas flight offered them a ride to Morgantown. At nearly midnight, an exhausted Carl was safely delivered to the home of Dean Bachmann, and Carl secretly worried about whether he could ever get back to New York.

Carl Malanga arrived at West Virginia University on July 1, 1970, with an academic rank of assistant professor of pharmacy. According to Carl, "Nineteen seventy was an exciting time in pharmacy. Ray Bachmann was rebuilding the WVU faculty and making plans for improvements in the direction that national education was going. That was the beginning of an emphasis on clinical pharmacy." Carl was hired to develop a two-semester sequence in therapeutics to accompany the clinical pharmacy emphasis in the curriculum. These courses were a departure from the basic course in pharmacology being taught at that time. The School had only a few clinical faculty (Pharm.D.s), about eight basic scientists, and two pharmacy-administration faculty. They worked very hard to develop a new curriculum and establish research laboratories, which until then were non-existent. "Dean Bachmann engendered interest in the faculty to do research and got the young faculty very much involved. Although this was quite strenuous, it was a labor of love." [9]

Ray Bachmann also wanted to introduce the newly acquired faculty to the state of West Virginia and its pharmacists. Discussing Ray Bachmann's method of doing so, Carl explained, "You haven't lived until you spent a Tuesday night with Ray Bachmann in his Pontiac Firebird, driving down Route 92 to Elkins for a four-county pharmacy society meeting and continuing education presentation by the new faculty member. Then, to drive back to Morgantown at 2 AM through a fog with ten feet of visibility was an experience not easily forgotten." One of the first pharmacists Carl met in Morgantown was Ann Dinardi (see Chapter 12), who leaned over and quietly told him, "Don't leave here. West Virginia has nice people and you'll like it here." Now decades later, Carl still remembers that admonition. He stayed until he retired, and both he and his wife Mary Lou loved West Virginia. They now live in South Carolina.

Following Ray Bachmann's untimely death (see Chapter 7), Dr. Louis Luzzi was hired as dean. During Dean Luzzi's tenure, several major changes occurred, one of which was to establish divisions in the school headed by coordinators. At that time, Dean Luzzi appointed Carl Malanga the coordinator for Basic Sciences. Shortly thereafter, Luzzi implemented the next phase of his plan to improve the graduate program. To meet the needs of both the professional and the graduate curriculum (e.g., offer a Ph.D. program in the Basic Pharmaceutical Sciences and Administrative and Behavioral Pharmacy), the School would have to departmentalize. The 1970s brought major changes with the formation of three departments and growth in the School's faculty size. While departmentalization offered many positives from the standpoint of administration and evaluation, it also created a degree of competition. Instead of being "one big happy family," Carl concludes there were now three families of "sometimes happy departments."

Carl was an excellent teacher who was highly respected by his students, as evidenced by his receipt of the School of Pharmacy Outstanding Teacher Award on 13 occasions. In 1994, Carl received a West Virginia University Foundation Award for University-wide outstanding teaching. For many years, he was also editor of the *Showglobe*. Carl retired September 30, 2002, after 32 years of exemplary service to West Virginia University. He was granted professor emeritus status effective October 1, 2002.[9]

In addition to the five faculty already mentioned, two deans have likewise been honored with emeritus status: Sidney Alan Rosenbluth and George R. Spratto. However, three other faculty, including one dean, fully met the criteria of emeritus faculty but their tenure at the West Virginia University School of Pharmacy preceded the origin of the official title. One of those individuals was Gordon Bergy.

Gordon Alger Bergy (also see Chapters 1, 5, 7 and 10) was born May 1, 1890, in Caledonia, Michigan. He graduated from the University of Michigan with a Ph.C. (Pharmaceutical Chemist) degree in 1913, following which he received a Bachelor of Science degree in 1915 and a Master of Science degree in 1916 from the same institution. His areas of expertise were food and drug chemistry, microbiology, vaccines and serum therapy. He joined

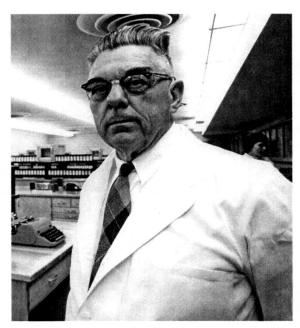

Professor Bergy in Laboratory

the faculty of the Department of Pharmacy of West Virginia University as its second member. Mr. Bergy and Dr. Rogers, the Department's founder, developed the curriculum. Soon thereafter, Dr. Rogers left the University, leaving Bergy as the sole Department member. In 1918, Bergy was called to active duty in the U.S. Army Chemical Warfare Service and the Department of Pharmacy closed. Bergy was subsequently furloughed to the West Virginia University ROTC unit in 1919. He served as head of the Department of Pharmacy from 1919 until 1936, when it separated from the School of Medicine to become the College of Pharmacy. As an undergraduate student, Professor Bergy was elected to membership in the Rho Chi Pharmaceutical Honorary Society and Phi Lambda Upsilon Honorary Chemical Society. As a faculty member, he was a contributing editor of *The American Professional Pharmacist* and had many scientific publications. In 1957, Professor Bergy was honored as a recipient of the WVPA's Dr. James Hartley Beal Award. Three years later on the occasion of his retirement with 44 years of service to the School and University, the alumni of the School of Pharmacy celebrated Gordon A. Bergy Day. That evening, 290 of his former students and fellow faculty attended the annual alumni banquet held in his honor.

However, some best remember Professor Bergy for his manner of dress. Always meticulously attired in a three-piece suit with a starched white shirt and tie, his shoes were often covered with mud. Bergy's garden, particularly his roses, were his pride and joy and a most important part of his life. He inspected his garden each morning before leaving home for the University. If his shoes were not muddied from the garden, mud was usually acquired on the walk to Woodburn Circle. Although he usually gave students a two-chapter reading assignment on the previous class day, his lecture on medicinal chemistry was contemplated *en route* to the University campus. Should insects be detected in his garden, the choice of chemicals to eradicate them might be incorporated into his lecture. If chapters on zinc and manganese were assigned for the next day's class, Bergy might instead lecture on the Haber process for the manufacture of ammonia, brought to mind as he walked by the DuPont plant en route to the University. Bergy's experience in chemical warfare during World War I accounted for one lecture each year on smoke, phosgene and chlorine gas. Little correlation could be found between class assignments and lectures, and only heaven knew what questions the examination would bring. In one lecture, Bergy admonished the students to remember what chemical could be used to remove a certain type of carpet stain. Bergy prefaced these remarks with, "Some day a woman will enter your pharmacy and ask how to remove this stain, and you will not remember the answer." Years later, a former student was asked that very question. With an astonished expression on his face, he paused to recall the answer, proffered the advice, and added, "Seven years ago Professor Bergy said some day I'd be asked that question, but I never dreamed it would take this long." He was convinced the woman thought he was weird. The Bergy Lecture, still held annually to bring distinguished pharmacy faculty to the School of Pharmacy, is a reminder of Professor Bergy's contributions to the School.

With respect to being fastidious and meticulous, Professor Bergy could not differ more than Professor Geiler; they were polar opposites. For example, as previously mentioned Professor Geiler meticulously measured out the alcohol in his compounding laboratory. Bergy, on the other hand, would place a quart of grain alcohol on the counter for student use. "Purple Jesus," a concoction of grape juice and alcohol consumed at many a fraternity party, was often provided courtesy of Professor Bergy's laboratory.

Despite his erratic teaching methods, many of his former students felt they learned more from Professor Bergy than from any other faculty member of the School of Pharmacy. Professor Bergy died November 23, 1966, in West Virginia University Hospital at the age of 76.

Dean Joseph Lester Hayman merits consideration for emeritus status along with Deans Rosenbluth and Spratto. Despite his years of service to

West Virginia, the pharmacy profession, and the School of Pharmacy, Dean Hayman died a decade prior to the origin of the emeritus award. His many contributions are documented in Chapters 3, 7, 10 and 11.

The last early faculty member deserving of emeritus status was Al Wojcik (also see Chapter 11). Upon graduation from the WVU School of Pharmacy in 1943, Albert Freddie Wojcik, born May 30, 1920, accepted a

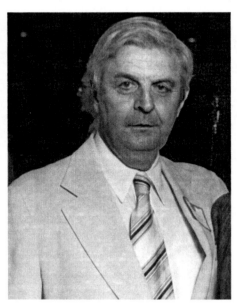

position with the Hoge Davis Drug Company in Wheeling, the city of his birth. However, the three-man faculty at the WVU School of Pharmacy at that time had need for expansion. Al, who graduated with the highest honors in his class and was an elected member of the Phi Lambda Upsilon chemistry honor society, was recruited. His credentials were impeccable. Al joined the faculty as an instructor in pharmacy in 1945.

As World War II ended, enrollment in the School of Pharmacy escalated, overwhelming the now four-man faculty in

Dr. Albert Freddie Wojcik

Morgantown. Veterans of World War II, taking advantage of the "G.I. Bill" to fund their education, swelled the ranks of the undergraduate student body. Due to the decline in enrollment during the war, only three students graduated from the WVU School of Pharmacy in 1945, a number that increased twelve fold by 1951. Having acquired only a bachelor's degree, Al needed graduate training to sustain his faculty status but could not be spared to enroll as a full time graduate student. His solution was to enroll part-time at the graduate school of the University of Pittsburgh School of Pharmacy for night classes during the winter months and as a full-time student in the summer.

Obtaining a master's degree did not go smoothly for Al. His wife, Louise, recalls a winter night when he had not returned from Pittsburgh by midnight. Louise called the State Police, worried he may have been involved in an accident. When Al finally arrived home in the early morning hours, she learned his car had skidded on a slick road and collided with a fire hydrant. Fortunately for Al he escaped injury, but the automobile was badly damaged.

Another minor "bump in the road" to his education had a somewhat better outcome. One of his professors at the University of Pittsburgh suddenly resigned and left the University without notifying Al. Al traveled to Pittsburgh to take the final examination in his course only to learn the professor had gone. Another faculty member, realizing Al's predicament, tested Al so he could receive the credit he deserved. This was an occasion when Al's Polish heritage may have been to his advantage: both Al and the altruistic professor shared the same ethnicity. Al was promoted to assistant professor of pharmacy in 1949 and received his Master of Science in pharmacy degree from the University of Pittsburgh in 1954. He then embarked on a path to obtain a Ph.D. in pharmacy administration. On receipt of his doctorate in 1970, he was promoted to professor of pharmacy administration.

Louise Wojcik relates an anecdote Al told her about Carl Furbee, Jr., an alumnus of the class of 1952.[10] One day Carl failed to show for class. Al knew the student's father, who would not countenance Carl skipping class very well. Knowing where Carl lived, Al went to his Sunnyside area residence and knocked on the door. When Carl answered he was stunned to find his professor there to inquire about his health. This action was typical of Al; he wanted his students to take full advantage of the education process to become better pharmacists. Louise adds, "Al was an example of the University's attitude of responsibility for student welfare…WVU is a family school and always has been." Another alumna, Ann Bond Smith, recalled Al's love for athletics. Every Saturday during football season he could be found taking tickets at the stadium gate near Martin Hall or at the old Field House at basketball games. "He always seemed to enjoy himself, chatting with alumni and friends when they returned for athletic events."[4]

Although students frequently complained about the lack of space when the School of Pharmacy was located in the basement of Woodburn Hall, Al never discussed these discomforts with his wife. When the Health Sciences Center was under construction, faculty were encouraged to visit other universities, such as the schools of pharmacy at The Ohio State University, University of Maryland and University of Pittsburgh, to learn about their classroom and laboratory arrangements to enhance WVU's teaching capabilities. Al made several such trips and provided a number of recommendations for design modifications for the new building.

Albert F. Wojcik retired from the faculty in his 40th year of teaching in 1984. For many years prior to his retirement, he served as editor of the School of Pharmacy *Showglobe*. He also served as alumni coordinator, a position he loved, and worked closely with the School's Alumni Association. With Al's leadership, the Alumni Association became one of the largest and most active alumni groups within the University community. Attendance at the annual pharmacy alumni banquet in those days frequently numbered between 200 and 300 graduates. In recognition of his work as alumni coordinator, the University presented Al with its Outstanding Service Award in 1974 and named him the 1977 Outstanding Alumnus. His interest in teaching and service to the University were widely recognized. He taught pharmaceutical jurisprudence, acted as a consultant on pharmacy law to the WV Board of Pharmacy, and helped prepare the law portion of the pharmacy licensure examination. Recognizing Al's service to the Board of Pharmacy, the University, and particularly to the WVPA, in 1981 the WVPA presented Al with the Dr. James Hartley Beal Award. In addition, the WVPA awarded Al its 1984 Board of Governors award for "meritorious service to the profession of pharmacy." Al was faculty advisor to Lambda Kappa Sigma for many years, a professional pharmacy fraternity whose goal is to promote women in pharmacy. For a decade following his retirement in 1984, an annual law lecture was given at the University to honor Professor Wojcik. Albert F. Wojcik died January 20, 1998. A few years prior to his death an *ad hoc* committee of School faculty was formed to consider awarding Al emeritus status. The work of that committee never came to fruition. To this day, an explanation for this omission remains a mystery.

Although they spanned the life of the School from its very beginning to recent times, the emeritus faculty shared other characteristics beyond their years of faithful service. Their love and respect for students were paramount. They actively sought and won students' respect. They were often groundbreakers, whether it involved developing a new curriculum, program, or coursework, reaching out to enhance alumni relationships or providing service to the university, community, state or nation. They persevered despite whatever obstacles their unique point in history presented to them, and they should be remembered for their many and diverse contributions to the profession and to the School of Pharmacy.

Part Four
Professional Leadership

Chapter Nine
The National Scene

Four West Virginia pharmacists have served as presidents of the American Pharmaceutical Association (now American Pharmacists Association) during three different eras. Three West Virginia pharmacists have presided over the National Association of Boards of Pharmacy in the same time frame. Two of these individuals, Roy Bird Cook and Newell Stewart, served as president of both organizations. Each was representative of his time, and all five were successful in their leadership role. Beyond that, there was little similarity among these individuals, particularly with regard to personality and leadership style.

Roy Bird Cook was born in a two-story log house in Roanoke, West Virginia, on April 1, 1886, the eldest of eight children. His home was located only four miles from the boyhood home of Confederate General Thomas J. "Stonewall" Jackson, which undoubtedly influenced his interest in history.[1] Educated in a public high school, he was one of only ten students in his class of 32 who graduated. They were further disappointed when commencement exercises were cancelled due to an outbreak of smallpox.[2]

Fascinated by the "mysteries of the drug store," Roy decided to become a pharmacist rather than follow in the footsteps of his newspaper editor father. At age 13, he was apprenticed to Minter B. Ralston at the Ralston and Bare Drug Store (founded in 1856) in Weston. Unable to attend a college level pharmacy program presumably due to his age, Roy enrolled in the Pharmaceutical Era Course on Pharmacy, a home study program designed

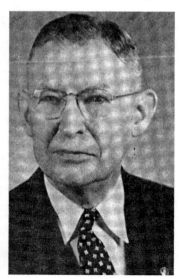

Roy Bird Cook

by Dr. James Hartley Beal, then president of Scio College of Pharmacy in Ohio. After grading his examination, Dr. Beal wrote "...your examination grade is 96% and I have recommended you for graduation."[3] Following a six-year apprenticeship, at age 19 Roy took the licensure examination and became licensed to practice pharmacy in West Virginia.[4]

Two years later Roy bought an interest in the store where he had trained and the pharmacy name was changed to Ralston and Cook, Druggists.[3] That same year he married and in 1909, the couple moved to Huntington where Roy practiced for ten years. Following a move to Charleston, Roy practiced with noted West Virginia pharmacist Arch Kreig, a former president of the West Virginia Pharmaceutical Association. Arch Kreig had a profound influence on young Roy, causing him to develop an interest in organized pharmacy that would persist throughout his professional life.

Over the next 30 years, Roy served the profession of pharmacy in various capacities. Initially appointed to the West Virginia Board of Pharmacy by a Republican governor in 1925, Roy, a Republican, was subsequently reappointed six of seven times by Democratic governors. He was elected secretary of the Board in 1932 and five years later in a national election became president-elect of the National Association of Boards of Pharmacy (NABP). Roy subsequently served as its president in 1938-39.

Interestingly, Roy's initial appointment to the West Virginia Board of Pharmacy came as a surprise to him. His partner in pharmacy practice at the time was Othor O. Older, whose term on the Board of Pharmacy was about to expire. Roy decided to meet with then Governor Gore to lend support to Older's reappointment to the Board. However, when the appointment was announced, it was Roy B. Cook rather than O.O. Older who was appointed to the Board. Roy and Othor's partnership subsequently dissolved.

In addition to his Board of Pharmacy activities, Roy served as secretary of the West Virginia Pharmaceutical Association and chair of the House of Delegates of the American Pharmaceutical Association (APhA). He was elected president of the American Pharmaceutical Association in 1942-1943. All of Dr. Cook's hard work did not go unrecognized. In 1949, he received the West Virginia Pharmaceutical Association's top award, the Dr. James H. Beal Award. In 1955, he received his greatest honor, the APhA's Remington Honor Medal, the nation's award for a pharmacist that is awarded annually in honor of Joseph Price Remington.[3,4,5] Dr. Cook is the only West Virginian to receive this prestigious award. When he presented Dr. Cook with the Remington Honor Medal, Dr. Robert L. Swain, a past president of the American Pharmaceutical Association, recognized Roy for his outstanding service as secretary of the West Virginia State Board of Pharmacy, his national service rendered to the profession in various capacities, and his relationship with other professions and the public.

However, those who knew Dr. Cook would probably ask the question, "which was his greatest passion, pharmacy or history?" Although he achieved national prominence as a pharmacist, Roy was equally renown as a civil war historian. In fact, during his presentation of the Remington Medal to Roy, Dr. Swain equated the qualities essential for a good historian to those same qualities required of a pharmacist. "Each," he said, "must be accurate, precise, and factual in his treatment of epoch-making events, world movements, and in his reading of records...The pharmacist must avoid error in his professional activities. His judgment must be sound and his interpretation of the prescription must...be infallible!"[6] These qualities were paramount for and characteristic of Dr. Cook. Roy authored many books and papers, including *Washington's Western Lands*, *The Family and Early Life of Stonewall Jackson*, and *Lewis County and the Civil War*. Additionally, shortly before his death, he had published *Lewis County and the Spanish-American War, Annals of Ft. Lee, Lewis County Journalists and Journalism,* and a history of the Christ Church Methodist. For the profession he is fondly remembered for his history of pharmacy published in 1946, *The Annals of Pharmacy in West Virginia.*

Dr. Cook served with distinction on the West Virginia Commission on Historic Scenic Markers, West Virginia War History Commission, and the Charleston Commission for Celebration of the 200th Anniversary of the Birth of George Washington. Historical papers and civil war letters collected by Roy Bird Cook have been gathered and catalogued in the West Virginia University Library. The Roy Bird Cook Collection contains eyewitness reports of many of the battles of the Civil War, personal letters of General Thomas J. "Stonewall" Jackson, and maps of Virginia and West Virginia antedating more than 250 years.

Dr. Cook has been honored by West Virginia University on three occasions: as a recipient of one of WVU's highest awards, an honorary Doctor of Laws degree; by having his papers, letters, and maps catalogued and published for others to enjoy and learn from; and by having the museum of the School of Pharmacy named the Cook-Hayman Museum in recognition of his accomplishments in pharmacy.[7]

His professional achievements might lead one to imagine Dr. Cook as a kind person, well liked by his colleagues and other associates. However, Dr. Cook had an authoritative, if not autocratic, attitude in dealing with his peers.

His demeanor differed from that of his former partner, Othor O. Older, who was described as "a lovely person, sweet and gentle who was universally loved by all who knew him." Such terms were not applicable to Dr. Cook. He was a stickler for detail and an individual "who would suffer no fools." However, Roy was also a masterful writer, a skill he undoubtedly inherited from his newspaper editor father. Few contemporaries could equal his use of the English language. In summary, Roy was a pharmacy leader in an era when those individuals were few in number but looked upon as giants in the profession. He started from humble beginnings and through perseverance and hard work rose to local and national recognition as a historian, historical writer, and pharmacy leader. For additional information about Roy Bird Cook, see Appendix D.

The second West Virginian who served as both president of the APhA and the National Association of Boards of Pharmacy was Sistersville native Newell W. Stewart (also see Appendix D). Born February 14, 1900, Newell served in the United States Army from 1918 to 1919 [8] and received a Ph.G. degree from the West Virginia University College of Pharmacy in 1923. As a student, he was elected into the Rho Chi honor society and after graduating, he practiced pharmacy for three years in Moundsville, West Virginia.

In 1926, however, young Newell opted for a warmer climate and moved to Phoenix, Arizona, where he operated a retail pharmacy for two decades. He served as secretary of the Arizona Board of Pharmacy and was a mayor of Phoenix before becoming president of the National Association of Boards of Pharmacy in 1948.[9] On assuming the NABP presidency, Newell found the issue of reciprocity remained an unsolved problem for NABP despite 40 years of debate. In his presidential address, he lamented the failure of the profession to enforce pharmacy laws and called upon the state boards to take immediate remedial action. Newell Stewart was an advocate for education and a strong proponent of establishing a pharmacy school at the University of Arizona. In 1947, he worked with the Arizona Board of Regents to obtain its approval and in 1949 the pharmacy school was separated from the University of Arizona College of Liberal Arts and became a full-fledged college. Newell receives much credit for the establishment of the University of Arizona College of Pharmacy and also served on its faculty during the early years.

Reflecting on his illustrious and productive career, the West Virginia University College of Pharmacy named Newell the 1953 recipient of its Outstanding Alumnus Award. Newell was elected president of the APhA in 1955.[8] During this time Newell contributed a number of articles to the *Journal of the American Pharmaceutical Association* regarding his vision for the future of the profession.[10] He likewise addressed this subject when West Virginia University selected Newell as the featured speaker at the 1955 Annual Banquet of the College of Pharmacy Alumni Association.[11] In his talk, Newell accurately predicted an era of more effective drugs that would enhance the quality of life and health of society. "Pharmacists," he opined, "by virtue of their education, will be viewed as equals by our allied professions." Stewart also called upon the West Virginia State Board of Pharmacy to oppose the state legislature that wished to consolidate the Board of Pharmacy with other boards, as had been recommended by the West Virginia Council of State Government at that time.

Newell believed there were three major problems for pharmacists in the 1950s that required remedial action by the profession: the escalation of health care costs, the lack of unity in the profession, and the need to police the profession. These issues remain problems today. Regarding the latter, he advocated stricter disciplinary action for ethics violations by pharmacists and insisted all pharmacists participate in reform. Newell retired after leaving office as APhA president in 1956. He remained active in the National Pharmaceutical Council until 1965. Newell died March 9, 1989, in Phoenix, Arizona.

The third West Virginian to serve as president of the APhA was David Stephen Crawford (also see Chapters 6 and 11 and Appendix D). A popular community pharmacist in Elkins, Steve served as president of the West Virginia Pharmaceutical Association in 1975-1976, and following a

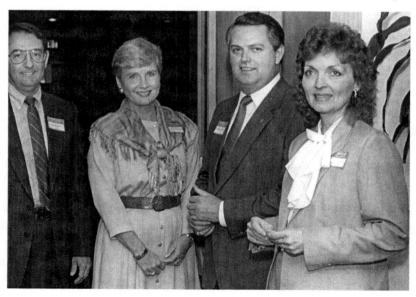

From right: Mrs. Crawford, Steve Crawford, Mrs. Riffee, Dean Bill Riffee
(University of Florida College of Pharmacy)

successful term in office, became president of the Academy of Pharmacy Practice in 1979-1980. In 1975, he formed Pharm-C Consultants, a group which employed pharmacists to provide "tailor-made" pharmacy services for small rural hospitals that would otherwise be unable to provide such services for their patients.[12] This unique enterprise garnered Steve national recognition, providing an opportunity for him to focus attention on the APhA. From 1981 to 1982, he served as speaker of the APhA House of Delegates and was elected president of the Association in 1987.

Stephen Crawford was also elected an International Pharmaceutical Federation community pharmacy section executive committee member.[13] He served on the West Virginia University School of Pharmacy Visiting Committee for more than two decades,[14] and in 1991, he was one of three pharmacists selected by the West Virginia State Legislature to serve on a joint House-Senate subcommittee to develop a new pharmacy reimbursement system for West Virginia. Having served his profession with distinction on both statewide and national levels, Steve returned to his roots and resumed community pharmacy practice in West Virginia. Steve unexpectedly died at his home in Elkins on May 19, 2007, after a brief illness. He led a productive life, serving both his profession and his patients well.

The most recent West Virginian to serve as president of the American Pharmacists Association (the Association name changed in 2003) was Thomas Edward Menighan (also see Chapters 10 and 11 and Appendix D) whose initial interest in pharmacy developed when given a chemistry set at age 11. A year later, he took a job in a local pharmacy in Sistersville and progressed up the chain from janitorial work to delivery boy to tending the soda fountain. As a pharmacy student, Tom was impressed by Dean Ray Bachmann's comment, "You're entering a profession where you'll never have to worry about making a living, so worry [instead] about making a difference." Menighan has remembered this sage advice throughout his years of pharmacy practice. He graduated *Cum Laude* in 1974, married his sweetheart, and accepted a position with a chain pharmacy located in Zanesville, Ohio. Having experienced this type of practice for four years and having been transferred a number of times, Tom purchased a Medicine Shoppe franchise and settled in Huntington, West Virginia, to start his own practice with Harvey Barton and Frank McClendon. Shortly thereafter, adversity took control of Tom's life. His wife was diagnosed with cancer that required extensive chemotherapy. One medical problem led to another. By necessity he became an expert in chemotherapy, home infusion therapy, and total parenteral nutrition (TPN).

Consumed by an entrepreneurial instinct, he formed a corporation called "Total Life Care" to provide home infusion services for West Virginia's two largest cities, Charleston and Huntington. Total Life Care began in a small back room of his Medicine Shoppe pharmacy. Extant today as Pharmacy Associates, Inc., this specialty-pharmacy and home care practice currently serves patients in 30 states. As a result of his successful practice, the APhA invited Tom to teach a short course on home infusion therapy and, impressed by his innovative teaching techniques, offered Tom an entry-level, management position in 1987.

During his first five years on the APhA staff, Tom advanced from Practice Management Associate to Director of State Affairs, and eventually to Senior Director of External Affairs. In the latter role, he was in charge of membership, public relations, state affairs, and new business development. From 1995 to 1998, he served on the APhA Board of Trustees and helped establish the Board's Finance Committee. In 2000, Tom was elected to a three-year term on the APhA board, serving as president of APhA the final year.[15, 16] Although Tom held the same position as his predecessor, Dr. Roy Cook, Tom's management style is markedly different. Whereas Dr. Cook was authoritative, Tom is a gregarious leader. Currently, Tom is general manager of Integrity Solutions, a division of Health Pathways, in the Washington, DC area. His company provides services and systems to pharmaceutical manufacturers, distributors, and pharmacies in the eastern United States.[16]

John Patrick Plummer was the third West Virginian to serve as president of the NABP, a position he held in 1983-1984. In the opening remarks of his presidential address, John stated that exactly 50 years had passed since Roy presided over NABP, and the NAPLEX examination was in its tenth year.[17] With the problem of reciprocity solved for 47 of the 50 states, John turned to what he considered the next most pressing problem, patient counseling. According to John, "Communication skills play a crucial role in assuring that patients receive appropriate drug information and we, therefore as Boards of Pharmacy, should encourage our registrants to develop these skills and apply them in counseling patients." He added, "The pharmacist has an excellent opportunity to test patients' recall of information

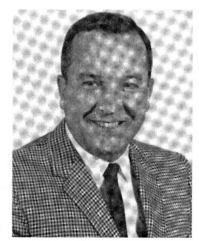

John Patrick Plummer

provided by the physician, to make the prescription instructions readily understandable, and to reinforce the patient's faith in prescribed therapy." [18]

John felt that NABP had been remiss in not addressing the improvement of practice by cooperating with state and national agencies. Turning to Article II of the NABP Constitution, John recalled: "The purpose of the Association is to provide for interstate reciprocity in pharmaceutic license, based upon a uniform minimum standard of pharmaceutic education and uniform legislation; to improve the standards of pharmaceutical education, licensure and practice *by cooperating with State, National, and International agencies and associations having similar objects.*" He suggested a central committee be formed with representatives from FDA, DEA, and NABP to discuss proposed regulations BEFORE they became law, rather than the current practice of the FDA enacting the laws for NABP to enforce.[19] Plummer's major concern was related to the FDA's practice of directly switching prescription drugs to over-the-counter (OTC) status. Plummer was one of many who believed the FDA bows to external demand, since the agency had recently switched numerous drugs from prescription to OTC status without prior notice. Plummer felt the FDA placed too much reliance on the consumer's ability to read and understand the product label. At that time with 44% of all OTCs distributed through grocery, convenience, or discount stores, Plummer felt the consumer was at considerable risk for adverse drug reactions. Fresh in Plummer's mind was the Alupent debacle, which followed the FDA's switching of prescription Alupent to OTC status without prior notice to the profession. Plummer advocated creating a third class of drugs, an "Exempt Legend Drug" category, that would restrict the sale of drugs in this class to the "hands-on" expertise of a registered pharmacist. FDA did not agree, and this drug category was never given a serious trial. The concept appeared to have died with Plummer's death in 2004. Nearly a quarter of a century after Plummer's address, in 2007 the Food and Drug Administration announced it is considering a "behind the counter" system that would permit greater consumer access to prescription drugs. In a *Wall Street Journal* article, the agency announced a hearing to explore the "public health benefit of drugs being available without a prescription but only after intervention by a pharmacist."[19] This intervention by a pharmacist is in keeping with the spirit of Plummer's presidential address.

These five West Virginians lived and practiced in different times and provided services for vastly different populations. However, all were pharmacy owners and each in his own way was an educator. They served their profession well, with a common interest and devotion to organized pharmacy.

Chapter Ten

The Local and
Regional Scene

The Early Years

West Virginia was the fourth state in the nation to organize a state association of pharmacists. The first West Virginia Pharmaceutical Association was formed in 1870 but did not survive. Regrettably, no record of this long forgotten first organization of pharmacists exists today.[1]

The Board of Commissioners of Pharmacy, antecedent to the Board of Pharmacy, advocated the formation of a professional organization open to all West Virginia "druggists." The Board was a self-supporting body with the authority to levy fines and collect fees. In effect, passage of the "Pharmacy Law of 1881" created the second West Virginia State Pharmaceutical Association by specifying that all monies collected by the commissioners were to be divided between that group and a yet to be formed state pharmaceutical association. The source of revenue lent impetus to the formation of this new association. Copies of the new pharmacy law were mailed to all known West Virginia pharmacists along with notice of an organizational meeting to be held in Wheeling on June 1, 1881. About a hundred druggists responded to the call, at which time a constitution was adopted for the new association. Samuel Laughlin, a Wheeling drug wholesaler whose family became prominent in the rapidly growing steel industry of that city, was selected as president of the meeting. Then Governor Jacob Jackson spoke to the assembly and discussed "some imperfections" in the Law of 1881. In particular, he noted that drug stores were regulated and restricted with regard to their sale of laudanum (an alcoholic preparation of opium) and other narcotics, and physicians who sold drugs were also subjected to the regulations and restrictions of the pharmacy law. However, no such restrictions were placed on the general public, meaning that a blacksmith or a grocer could sell narcotics without any legal ramifications. Amendments to correct these deficiencies were drafted at this meeting although not enacted.

The West Virginia State Pharmaceutical Association met yearly for the first several years but interest gradually waned and, after the 1885 meeting in Grafton, the organization disbanded. No doubt transportation difficulties in the largely rural state contributed to its demise. For the next 21 years, West Virginia languished without a pharmacy organization other than the Board of Commissioners. Then in 1906, Dr. James Hartley Beal used his masterful organizational abilities to help create the third state Association. Mr. S. Alfred Walker was named its first president.

Stephen Alfred Walker of Sutton, West Virginia, was born in Bloomville, Ohio. His older brother was also a pharmacist. Alfred had trained as

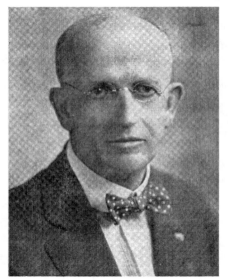

Stephen Alfred Walker

an apprentice in a drug store in Bettsville, Ohio, and in his brother's pharmacy in Kenton, Ohio. Prior to his apprenticeship he enrolled in Northwestern Ohio Normal School (currently Ohio Northern University) in Ada, Ohio, for a brief general education.[2] Mr. E.L. Juergens who operated a pharmacy in Sutton, West Virginia, recruited Walker to join his practice in 1891. Registered by the West Virginia Board of Pharmacy in 1892, Walker and Juergens renamed the firm "Juergens and Walker Drug Store." In 1901, Governor Albert B. White appointed Alfred Walker to the Board of Commissioners of Pharmacy. The following year Alfred was elected secretary of the Board of Pharmacy.

Alfred Walker met with Dr. Beal and the other invited druggists at Parkersburg's Chancellor Hotel in 1906 to organize the West Virginia State Pharmaceutical Association. Those 39 charter members included 10 future Association presidents. They approved a constitution, appointed Alfred as president, and decided to hold a yearly convention each June.

Alfred Walker gave his presidential address at the first annual Association convention on June 10, 1907. A half century later, Alfred's address was considered by those present to still be the best ever given at an Association meeting.[3] Alfred specifically laid out four goals of the fledgling organization: (1) to elevate the standard of pharmacy practice in West Virginia; (2) to protect the public; (3) to promote good fellowship among the members; and (4) to protect the interests of the profession by securing recognition and necessary legislation. He derived much pleasure from the successes of his year of Association leadership, which included the enactment of Dr. Beal's "new pharmacy law" by the state legislature; adoption of a constitution for the organization; identification of problems faced by West Virginia; and establishment of priorities for remedial action, most notably the unregulated sale of narcotics by merchants and the lay public. A remedy for this illogical law became Walker's first priority. Adding to Alfred's personal satisfaction was the enthusiasm of West Virginia pharmacists for their new organization, as evidenced by growth from the original 39 members to 186 active members in a mere nine months. Alfred was confident the West Virginia State Pharmaceutical Association (WVPA)[a] was built on a solid foundation and, unlike its predecessors, would now survive and flourish.

Alfred Walker's tenure as WVPA president was a resounding success. Well liked by his colleagues, he was a prosperous pharmacy owner who operated drug stores in both Sutton and Gassaway, West Virginia. After leaving office as president, he served as secretary of the Board of Pharmacy until his death in March 1932.[4] A civic minded individual, Alfred served on the City Council of Sutton and the Braxton County Board of Education. A highly successful businessman, he was president of the bank of Gassaway and a member of the Board of Directors for 25 years. He was made an honorary member of the Sutton Rotary Club, further attesting to the esteem in which he was held by his fellow citizens.[5] Active in the Republican Party he also served as chairman of the Braxton County Republican Executive Committee.

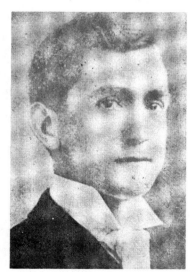

E. Bruce Dawson

Interestingly, the next two presidents of the WVPA, although born and reared as Ohioans, became staunchly loyal West Virginians. Ed Bruce Dawson was

[a] *The exact date the West Virginia State Pharmaceutical Association became the current West Virginia Pharmacists Association is unknown.*

registered to practice pharmacy in West Virginia on January 24, 1899, and despite living in Shadyside, Ohio, practiced in Wheeling. He was very active in the WVPA, serving as vice president from 1906 to 1907 and its second president from 1907 to 1908. During his administration, WVPA membership grew to 231 active and five honorary members. A handsome man, little is known about Bruce, who contributed so much to the WVPA. He continued active membership in the WVPA throughout his career. Despite living in Ohio where he also owned a pharmacy, Bruce never joined the Ohio Pharmaceutical Association, his allegiance remaining with the organization he once headed.[6] Neither his date of birth nor record of education survive. In 1925, Bruce moved to Cleveland where he practiced pharmacy until his death in October, 1946. His obituary in *The Cleveland Plain Dealer* merely listed his profession and the date of his death.

Another moving force in the formation of the WVPA was Arch Kreig from Logan, Ohio. An 1889 graduate of the Cincinnati College of Pharmacy, Arch was awarded a gold medal for graduating first in his class. Although his initial pharmacy practice was in Cincinnati, he moved to Charleston, West Virginia, in 1896 where he practiced for 57 years. Arch was the first secretary of the Association, a position he held for two years, and served again as secretary from 1911 to 1947. He served as its third president from 1908 to 1909. The first five presidents of the WVPA were all strong proponents for a pharmacy program at West Virginia University (WVU). A strong association, they reasoned, would enhance membership recruitment and invigorate their peers, and a teaching program in Morgantown at WVU would augment both. Their confidence in success was confirmed at the 1909 convention in Morgantown. Then WVU President, Dr. D.B. Purinton, gave the welcoming address, which was responded to by WVPA President-elect William W. Irwin. A resolution favoring the founding and maintenance of a School of Pharmacy in connection with the University was drawn up and read to the membership by Weston pharmacist Stephen T. Tierney.[7] It supported the position of the "five founding fathers" of the fledgling WVPA organization and was readily adopted without dissent. At that meeting, the Committee on Legislation also reported success in prohibiting the sale of poisons by persons other than pharmacists along with a provision that only a registered pharmacist could fill a prescription. President Arch Kreig recommended abolition of the statewide tax of $25.00 per drug store, believing that pharmacists' work should not be taxed to support the

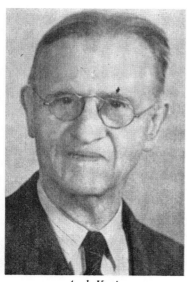

Arch Kreig

general government fund. Treasurer W.S. Vinson reported the Association was in "a prosperous condition of affairs."

The second day of the convention provided a scientific session for the assembled pharmacists. Professor A.R. Whitehill of WVU delivered "an interesting lecture on electricity that was well received by the audience which showed their appreciation by paying the closest attention and applauding at the conclusion of the lecture." Professors J.H. Beal of Scio College and John Uri Lloyd, a Cincinnati pharmacist and professor of chemistry at the Eclectic Medical Institute at Worthington, Ohio, also gave scientific addresses. It did not go unnoticed that despite being an Ohio resident, Professor Beal had attended each convention since the organization was formed. Entertainment on the final day of the convention included a baseball game for the men, a bowling tournament for the women, and an auto ride along the banks of the Cheat River.[7]

The life of the fourth founding father of the WVPA, William W. Irwin, revolved around two organizations: his fraternal lodge and his professional association. Irwin served in 1897 as Potentate of the Osiris Temple in Wheeling and in 1913 became Imperial Potentate of the Shriners of North America. Occupancy of such a lofty Masonic position brought William Irwin national recognition, equal to, if not greater than, that of noted West Virginia pharmacist leaders Roy Bird Cook and J. Lester Hayman. His pharmacy, it was said, "was a gathering place for Masons and Democrats." However, Irwin assumed the presidency at an ideal time since his commitments to masonry were ending as pharmacy's needs were on the rise. William S. Vinson succeeded Irwin as the fifth WVPA President (1910 to 1911). He became nationally known as a founder of the National Association of Retail Druggists (now National Community Pharmacists Association). Few states can boast of a more illustrious team of early leaders than WVPA's "founding five."

The convention held in Webster Springs, West Virginia, on July 17-19, 1911, has been described as a "lively one," although the term "contentious" would perhaps be more appropriate. West Virginia grocers were still selling narcotics and would not give up their lucrative business without a fight.

Four bills regarding narcotics that were grocer-supported were pending in the state legislature, although the Association's influence prevailed and each was defeated. Likewise, a major struggle ensued to defeat the West Virginia "Coca Cola Bill," intended to license the sale of that famous beverage that was gaining popularity. A resolution was also adopted urging defeat of the "Patent Medicine Tax Stamp Bill" pending in the U.S. Congress.

Past President E. Bruce Dawson presented a paper discussing "The Advantages of a School of Pharmacy at the State University," and a committee consisting of the Association's officers was appointed to meet with University officials to discuss plans for a pharmacy school in Morgantown. Finally, pharmacists celebrated their victory in the legislature of a reduction in their license fee from $25.00 to a mere $2.00.

The president elected at the 1911 WVPA Convention was cut from a different mold than his predecessors. George Orville Young, of Buckhannon, West Virginia, known to his friends as "G.O.," was born in Fairmont, West Virginia, and graduated from Scio College in 1896 with a Ph.G. degree. His father was a Methodist minister who provided him with a devoutly religious background. G.O. first practiced four years in Cumberland, Maryland, then became a sales representative for the William S. Merrell Company (now Sanofi-Avantis) and traveled through West Virginia for three years. In 1902, he purchased a pharmacy in Buckhannon and filled the first prescription in his new pharmacy on September 15, 1902. Seven years later, he was elected secretary of the WVPA and served in that capacity for two years prior to assuming its presidency.

North central West Virginia was sparsely populated in the early 1900s and a pharmacist could expect a modest income at best. To enhance his income, G.O. added a wholesale pharmacy to his store with disappointing results. He erected a new building to house his pharmacy and heavily invested to make it as physically attractive as possible. He personally designed the soda fountain, which was built to order in Pittsburgh, along with an ice cream plant unlike any other in the region. G.O. didn't merely make ice cream; rather, he insisted, "I manufactured it." Years later he would tell friends a favorite anecdote that occurred early one Sunday morning. A party of four men appeared before the usual opening time and knocked on the pharmacy door. The clerk had not yet arrived and George was alone in the store. Aware that the visitors had seen him, George admitted the four men who requested ice cream sodas that George obligingly made for them. One of the customers then asked for a sandwich, to which George responded with directions to a near-by restaurant. Somewhat miffed, the customer queried, "What kind of a drug store is this?" Although George's response is not known, he later learned the identity of his customers that Sunday morning. They were Harvey Firestone, Henry Ford, Thomas A. Edison and John Burroughs, the noted author and poet. He never saw the four of them again.[8]

George soon realized that the commercial property and casualty insurance then available to the small businessman was prohibitively expensive. When he completed his year at the helm of WVPA, his entrepreneurial instinct kicked in and, with a small group of fellow pharmacists, organized the American Druggists' Fire Insurance Company, later known as the American Druggists' Insurance Company of Cincinnati, Ohio. G.O. Young not only provided low cost insurance coverage for his fellow druggists, he created a company unique in the insurance industry, one that understood the pharmacy profession. As the years passed, American Druggists' provided fire and casualty insurance to pharmacies in 41 states at a cost affordable for the rural independent pharmacist.[8] G.O. was vice president of the American Druggists' Company for its first 20 years, and served on its board of directors until his death at the age of 85. During G.O. Young's year as Association president, an unrelated but interesting incident occurred. Arch Tetrick was an individual who had applied for a pharmacy license in Blacksville, WV. Unfortunately for Arch, the Board of Pharmacy summarily rejected it. Being young and lacking an established reputation, Tetrick was perplexed by this disapproval. Upon investigation, Tetrick learned the Woman's Christian Temperance Union was the culprit that had opposed his license, fearing young Arch might sell liquor in his pharmacy. Years before another druggist in that locality had sold liquor, an action that was unacceptable to the Temperance Union membership. Arch resolved the problem through personal diplomacy and ultimately obtained his license.

Little information exists about the presidents during the next five years. Later in that decade, as the world became engulfed in a war Woodrow Wilson assiduously avoided as "Europe's conflict," a modest and affable pharmacist from Putnam County, West Virginia, was elected the 12th president of WVPA. Othor O. Older (also see Chapter 10) had an inauspicious beginning in pharmacy to match his rather unusual name. Enrolled in the University of Cincinnati College of Pharmacy, he dropped out of school after his first year. After leaving school, he purchased half interest in M.J. Browning and Company, a Charleston pharmacy that he renamed Browning and Older. Later, he returned to Cincinnati and received a Ph.B. degree in 1901. The following year he purchased the remainder of Browning and Older that he renamed Older Drug Company. From 1926 to 1944, he practiced with Mr. Roy Bird Cook in a practice known as Older-Cook Drug Company. Mr. Older left that practice in 1944 for a solo practice in Charleston from which he retired six years later.

Othor was president of WVPA from 1917 to 1918. Association activity was curtailed during the war years due to the large number of pharmacists in the military. No convention was held in 1918; instead, a meeting to conduct the business of the Association and to select officers for the following year was held in Charleston. Roy Bird Cook was elected to succeed Older as president from 1918 to 1919. Minutes of the meeting were not kept and only 25 members attended. The only speaker discussed war taxes and war stamps.

With the armistice concluding the First World War, annual conventions resumed with the 1919 convention held in Wheeling. John C. Davis, a relative newcomer to West Virginia, was then elected president of the Association. An associate of the Hoge-Davis Drug Company in Wheeling, little is known of this individual except that he sold his interest in the Hoge-Davis Company in 1921 and moved to Canton, Ohio. The State Attorney General addressed the membership at the 1919 convention regarding his interpretation of the Child Labor Law that prohibited children under age 16 from working in pharmacies beyond seven in the evening. Three resolutions were adopted by this convention: it was resolved to prohibit immigrants who were not naturalized citizens from being registered as pharmacists in West Virginia; it was further resolved to enforce the poison law prohibiting sale of poisons by retail grocers; and it was also resolved to endorse Woman's Suffrage. Professor Gordon A. Bergy, who had recently returned from service in the Army Chemical Corps, was elected treasurer of the WVPA at that time.

Between the Wars

By the 1920 convention, most pharmacists in the armed services had returned to civilian life and pharmaceutical education was of lesser concern to the conventioneers. It was announced that entrance requirements to the School of Pharmacy now required a four-year high school degree rather than the former prerequisite of only one year. Professor Gordon A. Bergy announced the addition of J. Lester Hayman to the faculty of the School to teach pharmacognosy. Mr. Charles E. Lively, West Virginia Director of Prohibition, spoke on the topic "The National Prohibition Law." Resolutions adopted by the convention that year urged better pay for university faculty (a perennial request by faculty), better care for drug addicts, a resolution to combine the association offices of treasurer and secretary, and an objection to the U.S. Army policy of not giving preference to pharmacists over non-professional applicants in the Medical Administrative Corps.[b] Of the four resolutions adopted, only that combining the office of WVPA treasurer and secretary was implemented.

Charles V. Selby, WVPA president in 1933 to 1934, was also a founder of the American College of Apothecaries (ACA) and a highly regarded member of both associations. Selby is credited with shaping the ACA during its first decade from 1940 to 1950 utilizing experience gained from his presidency of the WVPA. From 1940 to 1965, he missed only one meeting of the ACA, in 1944 during wartime, and all the while operated a community pharmacy in Clarksburg, West Virginia. He was elected the first secretary-treasurer of the ACA in 1940 and served in that office for a decade. The ACA had a spartan beginning. Mr. Selby's meager office equipment consisted of a typewriter, a stand, a storage closet and an addressograph machine. When a stenographer was hired in 1945, Selby commented the stenographer was "the only paid employee in the organization."[10]

A list of the WVPA presidents appears in Appendix E, but many of their stories have been lost to history. A descendant of one president wept when interviewed, happy that her long forgotten hero would now be remembered. Some, like Fred Watkins and Fred Allen, are still recognized for their service to the state of West Virginia in elective or appointive office. Bill Coleman, Charles Selby, and Othor Older are best recalled for their outstanding pharmacy practices and outgoing personalities.

Post War Years

It is unfortunate that few documents recording the achievements of WVPA presidents and their administrations from 1920 to 1950 survive. Sketchy records of only nine presidents from these three decades have been reconstructed, and no data regarding their administrations exist. Publication of a state pharmaceutical journal did not begin until 1948. However, in 1950, a small group of past presidents with more than a passing interest in the organization decided to form a club within the Association, which they called the Past Presidents Club. Minutes of this Club exist and provide insight into

---

[b] *The Medical Administrative Corps (MAC) was organized in 1921 and the Pharmacy Corps was organized in 1943. Public Law 80-337, 4 August 47, abolished MAC, the Sanitary Corps, and the Pharmacy Corps to create the Medical Service Corps.*

the workings of the WVPA during the years 1950 through 1989.

Virgil R. Hertzog, a past president himself, founded the Past Presidents Club to provide a venue by which the former WVPA presidents could continue their service to the organization in a problem solving capacity after leaving office. Although they could only make suggestions to the WVPA Council, the past presidents fervently believed that inherent laxness in the structure of the Association justified the Club's existence.[11] By 1955, the Past Presidents Club was well organized and thriving, and it began to evolve into an oversight committee for the Association. The past presidents possessed a wealth of experience and knowledge which often surpassed that of newly elected officers. Furthermore, Club members resided in almost every region of the state and collectively represented the profession as a whole. Even though the club was formed without an oversight purpose, there was an undeniable logic for that concept.[11]

Although the minutes and records from the Past Presidents Club generally reflected routine discussions or business, some humorous and rather astonishing events were recorded. In 1955, Fred McFarlin (St. Albans) opened the discussion at one meeting by suggesting wives be invited to attend future meetings. His suggestion was rejected on the basis that meetings were held strictly for business purposes and "wives should be excluded for the good of the Association."[12]

The poor quality of the Association's monthly journal, *The West Virginia Pharmacist*, was a principal concern voiced at the Club meeting in 1955. Roy Bird Cook complained the journal published little news worth reading, while another past president emphasized the paucity of space allotted by the editor for news items from the component local societies. In a representative issue of the journal (March 1955), 19 pages were devoted to advertising, six and a half pages to [free] publicity for pharmaceutical manufacturers, and only two pages were allotted for news items from the county societies. Roy Bird Cook reported that material being provided as news items to the secretary-manager/editor were not being published.[13] The secretary-manager, whose name has been purposely omitted, had been hired in 1955 by the Association for three specific purposes: to relieve the officers of administrative work, to visit pharmacies throughout the state to recruit new members, and to assume overall responsibility for the monthly journal. Ernest Hoge and G.O. Young felt the secretary-manager was derelict in his responsibility to increase enrollment in the state society and should "spend more time in the field" contacting non-member pharmacists and pharmacies.[13] In fact, no record of pharmacy visitations can be found. Membership in the organization had not increased since the secretary-manager had been hired while Association expenses were escalating. Most members of the WVPA had no knowledge of the Association's then financial status. Likewise, the former presidents did not fully appreciate the magnitude of the existing problems that were, in reality, a harbinger of impending disaster.

Why were expenses of the state Association escalating? Several factors were involved, none of which were common knowledge to the members. Association funds were being used to pay the secretary-manager's expenses in full to attend meetings. He attended the annual meetings of each of the near-by state associations, as well as the annual meetings of the major national pharmaceutical associations, such as APhA and NARD. Then, there was the matter of salary. The secretary-manager was paying himself a salary of $8,400 a year, compared to an average salary of $5,500 for a small rural community pharmacy owner.[14] Entertainment expenses at the annual conventions were also considerable, with entertainers brought in from New York and Florida rapidly depleting the treasury. No formal accounting of the Association budget had occurred since 1953. In 1958, Mr. Hertzog reported that for a third consecutive year the WVPA had operated at a loss, incurring a deficit of $1,777 that year. Again, membership recruitment was unsuccessful. The secretary-manager was not traveling around the state to recruit new members despite specific instructions to do so. Association members were unaware of these problems because minutes were not promptly distributed. This was not an attempt by Mr. Hertzog, who functioned as secretary for the meetings, to cover up the secretary-manager's ineptitude; rather Virgil had a single person pharmacy and lacked the time to be an effective secretary. Minutes were being transcribed from Hertzog's handwritten notes nearly a year after an annual meeting, resulting in incomplete and imprecise minutes in which concerns discussed were not being recorded.

The Past Presidents Club did not meet again until 1961 due to the death of G.O. Young, a driving force behind the Club. Interest in continuing the Past Presidents Club had reached a nadir. As a group, the former presidents lacked clout and were dependent upon the WVPA Council to initiate change. It now appears the WVPA, itself a victim of chronic fiscal instability, was in danger of falling apart. Little business was conducted at the 1961 Club meeting. The primary item of business at the 1962 meeting was to pass a resolution to increase pharmacists licensure fees to meet the needs of the

State Board of Pharmacy. No record of a Past Presidents Club meeting in 1963 exists. A financial bombshell was dropped one year later.

Mr. John P. Plummer of Fairmont, then incoming WVPA president, called a special meeting of the Club in September 1964 to apprise the members of the circumstances related to the secretary-manager's sudden departure from West Virginia two months earlier.[15] Subsequent to the secretary-manager's departure, Mr. Plummer and Fairmont attorney Tom White had flown to Florida where they met with the former secretary-manager. He "was advised that should he return to West Virginia he would face criminal prosecution on charges of embezzlement of funds from the Association." The secretary-manager complied and made no attempt to return to West Virginia.[15] No accounting of the amount of embezzlement survives to this date, although the loss was felt to be considerable and potentially in the tens of thousands of dollars.

Mr. John "Jack" H. Neale who was elected to the WVPA Council clearly recalled the events at that time. Mr. Neale had been trying to get "an independent audit of the secretary-manager's books for several years," but, according to Neale, "the secretary-manager was popular and had a number of powerful supporters. Secretary Hertzog and past presidents Lester Hayman, Bill Stuck, Joe Pugh (early on), and Roy Bird Cook were solidly behind the secretary-manager. With such strong support, it took some time to get a majority on the Council to support an audit….and it was the impending audit that resulted in his [sudden] departure."[16]

In retrospect, red flags to the possibility of an embezzlement appeared in the minutes of the Past Presidents Club for several years but were not fully appreciated.[17-20] The secretary-manager was described as the "fair-haired boy" of Dr. Roy Bird Cook, who wielded immense power by virtue of having been secretary of the Board of Pharmacy for three decades. Additionally, Dr. Cook was highly regarded nationally as a recipient of the prestigious Remington Medal.[21] Having a supporter of Dr. Cook's caliber, the secretary-manager was considered by many to be beyond reproach and therefore beyond accountability.[22] The secretary-manager had also been hired on the recommendation of J. Lester Hayman, dean of the West Virginia School of Pharmacy who was likewise a former past president. Having the support of the two most highly regarded members of the Association made the secretary-manager virtually untouchable.[21]

The Past Presidents Club was the first group to suspect something was amiss in the Association administration,[22] but proof was not easily obtained.

The former presidents met only once a year, following which they returned to their hometowns and practices leaving the secretary-manager unsupervised and unobserved over the next year. The Association appeared to have had no accountant or regular audits, a fact unknown to the membership who believed the WVPA was operating smoothly.

Who was ultimately to blame for the WVPA debacle? It is easy to point the finger at the secretary-manager since he merits the lion's share of the burden. However, despite having been highly recommended for the position, he lacked proper qualifications, for which the WVPA Council who hired him bears the responsibility. The Council not only failed to oversee the secretary-manager, but also overlooked the absence of regular audits. Dean Hayman accepted complete responsibility for the situation; although not truly his fault, he had initially referred the recent School of Pharmacy graduate to the Council with a laudatory recommendation. Secretary Hertzog also took a measure of responsibility for the nine-year delay in recognizing that the secretary-manager was dishonest. His meeting minutes were hopelessly garbled and vaguely written. His habit of delayed transcription resulted in a lack of continuity between meetings. On one occasion, Mr. Hertzog's handwritten notes were misplaced and transcribed two years later. Had transcriptions been promptly made, perhaps the secretary-manager's failures would have come to light sooner. As an example, the mundane search for a manufacturer to make a past president's lapel pin occupied as much space in the Association minutes as did its precarious finances. The WVPA membership must also share blame in this incident; it lacked a close supervisory capacity. At the close of a statewide convention, the unsupervised secretary-manager had a splendid opportunity to commit fraud.

According to Mr. Willard Phillips, the business consultant who replaced the secretary-manager as executive secretary in 1965, the response of the State's pharmacists to the depleted Association treasury was phenomenal.[23] Mr. A.F. "Sixty" Bond (Clendenin) and Mr. Harry Lynch (Charleston) stepped forward and took over as "temporary co-secretary-managers" to run the Association and its office until Mr. Phillips was hired.[24] Mr. Carl Furbee (Bridgeport), Mr. Jack Neale (Charleston), and Mr. John Plummer actually hired relief pharmacists to work in their pharmacies while they volunteered their time to the Association.[22, 24] Contributions of thousands of dollars were sent to the Association,[25] with generous supporters giving over $2,000 in just one evening to save the virtually bankrupt Association.[27] The money obtained supported the Association until dues could replenish the depleted treasury.[28] By 1968, indebtedness due to the former secretary-manager was reported to be only $3,250; it was optimistically expressed that another year would bring complete resolution.[29]

The Past Presidents Club held its last meeting on August 13, 1989, with only eight attendees. No major problems had required the Club's attention since the 1964 embezzlement, which the Club members helped to remedy. Finances had ceased to be a problem with proper management, and the WVPA appeared to be running smoothly. The conventions had changed from ones with lavish entertainment to those offering professional programs with notable speakers. Essentially, in its final 23 years the Past Presidents Club encountered no situations for which its expertise and wisdom were needed. Members' time was spent selecting candidates for WVPA's three awards, the Bowl of Hygeia Award, the Dr. James Hartley Beal Award, and the Outstanding Pharmacists Award.[28] Interest in the Past Presidents Club gradually dwindled as did meeting attendance.[30]

It was both ironic and fitting that the same pharmacist who conceived and organized the Past Presidents Club in 1950 was the one to dissolve the organization 39 years later. Mr. Virgil R. Hertzog "retired" from the club in August 1989. No meetings were scheduled thereafter.

A New World Develops

The Second World War resulted in a societal change not fully appreciated until many years later. Prior to 1940, most pharmacists and their clerks were male. By necessity, women replaced their male counterparts during the war as the former clerks entered the armed services. By 1946, the nation had nearly reverted to prewar status; however, male pharmacy clerks were gone forever. The demise of the male clerk was an unintended consequence of a brilliant plan concocted by the U.S. Congress for an entirely different purpose. To avoid formidable unemployment and economic disaster with the end of the war, a program was devised to absorb twelve million men from the armed services and gradually assimilate them back into society. Referred to as the "G.I. Bill," it provided educational opportunities for the bulk of the veterans. Provision of paid tuition, books, and subsistence for 36 months served as incentive for young veterans to obtain a college or trade school education to enhance their marketability in the workforce. Many of the prewar clerks took advantage of the "G.I. Bill" rather than return to their jobs. Some veterans enrolled in pharmacy schools and upon graduation helped eliminate the pharmacist shortage that existed at the war's end. A companion program designed for those less interested in pursuing advanced education was commonly known as the "52/20 Club." This provided veterans twenty dollars a week for 52 weeks, a significant sum of money at the time, provided they remained unemployed. The G.I. Bill was a resounding success, providing thousands of veterans (including many future pharmacists) who otherwise could not have afforded a college education with the chance to advance up the economic ladder. In contrast, the "52/20 Club" often served as a crutch for unmotivated veterans. Congress also provided a G.I. Bill (but not the 52/20 Club) following the Korean War, resulting in a workforce education level that was unsurpassed either before or since in American society.

Another change brought about by World War II was a gender shift. For the first 80 years of the WVPA's existence, each of its presidents was male. Over the decades from 1986 to 2006, six women were elected president (Appendix E). These women provided effective leadership for the Association and were themselves highly successful professionals. As the first female president of WVPA in 1986, Sandra Justice (also see Chapter 12) emphasized student involvement in the Association. Sandra created a venue in which students became active in WVPA, resulting in a positive image and other benefits for the Association. She and pharmacy student Jann Burks Skelton also facilitated WVU student involvement regionally and nationally in the APhA student organization (now known as the Academy of Students of Pharmacy). As a result of ongoing student leadership roles, West Virginia students have frequently won awards of excellence at APhA for patient care projects.

Debra Warden Nichol was elected president of WVPA at the 1987 convention. Debra was the second woman to hold this position with a stated goal of uniting the profession. Debra and her administration facilitated the passage of legislation requiring mandatory continuing education for pharmacists, promulgated physician-dispensing regulations, and literally revamped the organization. The reorganization included adding sections for community pharmacists, institutional practice pharmacists, and consulting pharmacists, a first effort by the WVPA to unify all aspects of pharmacy practice.

In 1992, Karen Reed followed in Debra's footsteps. Karen's administration recognized the need for a new Pharmacy Practice Act to govern the profession. At that time, pharmacy technicians were not legally recognized. Karen chaired a committee to rewrite the Act and shepherded it through passage two years later. Likewise, promotion of the Pharmacists

Recovery Network (PRN) was initiated during her administration. Karen thinks of her achievements as a professional reward of greater magnitude than any other she could possibly receive. Subsequently, Karen was elected a member of the APhA Board of Directors and became a national spokesperson of the organization for patient education by pharmacists.

Past President Carol Ann Hudachek's (president in 1995 to 1996) career has evolved differently from the previous female WVPA presidents in that her practice encompasses extensive teaching and education work. In addition to being the clinical pharmacy manager at Weirton Medical Center, Carol holds academic appointments at West Virginia Northern Community College and with the National Association for Practical Nurse Education and Service, Inc. (NAPNES) of Silver Spring, Maryland. Carol also holds clinical pharmacy preceptor appointments at the schools of pharmacy of Duquesne University, West Virginia University, University of Pittsburgh, and Ohio Northern University. Other activities Carol has been involved with include writing articles about drug use for area newspapers, operating a call-in radio program, and presenting numerous community educational programs.

Maribeth Nobles, WVPA president in 1999 to 2000, considers her administration's leading accomplishment to be the implementation of a strategic plan, one goal of which was to develop and maintain a membership and leadership base that was broadly representative of the pharmacy profession. By-laws were changed to enable the Board of Directors to better represent different practice areas. The organization's focus was redirected to include more pharmacy students and technicians. A second goal was to develop the financial resource base necessary for long-term success. The third goal was to achieve appropriate organizational changes to support strategic plan implementation. Membership e-mail addresses were compiled and plans were made for development of a website. The fourth goal was to develop and implement a strong legislative agenda. The final goal was to provide the membership with comprehensive continuing education programming. Maribeth worked as a staff pharmacist at the Veterans Administration Hospital in Martinsburg, West Virginia, where she became an integral factor in providing care for West Virginia's veterans.

Patricia Johnston (also see Chapter 12 and Appendix E) is another of the "new breed" of pharmacists. As an Association past president (2003 to 2004), Patty takes pride in her work with the West Virginia legislature for a collaborative practice bill. Patty's community pharmacy practice is located in Beckley, West Virginia, and focuses on diabetes and cholesterol management, health education, and fitness. Unique to her practice is a dietitian employed to provide dietary advice to her patients. Eighteen to 20 WVU pharmacy students a year complete experiential rotations at her pharmacy. In appreciation for her efforts, the West Virginia University School of Pharmacy recognized Patricia as the 2000 Preceptor of the Year and 2007 Co-Preceptor of the Year.

Of no lesser import over the past two decades has been the emergence of pharmacists as entrepreneurs, with past presidents Frank McClendon and Tom Menighan serving as striking examples of such individuals. Frank McClendon, who previously practiced with Tom in Huntington, has taken the provision of pharmaceutical services to an entirely new level in West Virginia. Frank McClendon excels in creative marketing and public communication. He has produced a series of 45-second radio vignettes that are utilized by pharmacies throughout the nation to promote drug-use compliance by educating the public about food-drug and drug-drug interactions involving over-the-counter medications. Frank is also chief operating officer of Comprecare, a corporation he formed to provide home infusion solutions and home medical and respiratory equipment to patients living in Ohio, Kentucky, and West Virginia. Comprecare also provides specialized therapy such as human growth hormone to patients in 32 states. Tom Menighan's accomplishments are discussed in Chapters 9, 11, and 13.

In summary, the presidents of the West Virginia Pharmacists Association were outstanding professionals who helped to meet the needs of their era in diverse ways. Many held national leadership roles. Others have unique practices or distinguished themselves as small chain owners beyond West Virginia's borders. Still others have served in or founded national professional organizations that likewise enhanced West Virginia's reputation. West Virginia can be justifiably proud of the contributions and leadership of these individuals.

Chapter Eleven
And the Winner is . . . WVPA Awards

The West Virginia Pharmacists Association (WVPA) presents four awards to recognize excellence in pharmacy practice by West Virginians. These awards are the biannual Dr. James Hartley Beal Honor Award, and the annually presented Bowl of Hygeia, Distinguished Young Pharmacist and Innovative Pharmacy Practice Awards. Many deserving and accomplished individuals have received these awards. The stories of several of these recipients follow.

The Beal Award is the oldest and most prestigious award presented by the WVPA, given in recognition of outstanding and meritorious service that furthers the interests of the pharmacy profession in West Virginia. First presented in 1947, it was named to honor Dr. James H. Beal, considered to be the "father" of the WVPA. Dr. Beal, born in 1861 in New Philadelphia, Ohio, earned a Ph.G. degree from the Scio College of Pharmacy in 1884 and a Bachelor of Laws degree from the Cincinnati School of Law in 1886. Dr. Beal became dean of the Scio College of Pharmacy the following year and served in that position until 1907.[1] Scio College, a one-program university, merged with Mount Union College in 1911 after a brief existence of only 54 years. Although Dr. Beal lived in Ohio, he had strong ties to West Virginia where many of his students resided. Dr. Beal utilized his legal expertise to help write the first West Virginia Pharmacy Practice Act in 1882 (see Chapter 1) and in so doing, created one of the nation's first boards of pharmacy. The WVPA established the following qualifications for the Dr. James Hartley Beal Honor Award:

1. Pharmacist licensed in West Virginia
2. Member of WVPA for at least 10 years and a resident of West Virginia
3. Evidence of meritorious service in furthering the interest of the profession of pharmacy in West Virginia

Past recipients of the Dr. James Hartley Beal Honor Award include individuals who have distinguished themselves in pharmacy practice, as well as pharmacists who have served as legislators, academicians or entrepreneurs. Due to their accomplishments, many of the Beal Honor Award winners have been discussed in other chapters, including Roy Bird Cook (second recipient, also see Chapters 1, 7, 9, 10 and Appendix F), George Orville Young (third recipient, also see Chapters 4, 10 and Appendix F), and

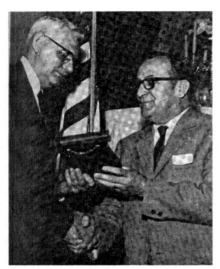

(Right to Left) Dean Bachmann Presenting Beal Award to Fred Geiler

Fred C. Allen (fifth recipient, also see Chapters 3, 4, 5, 10 and Appendix F). Academicians who received the Beal Honor Award include J. Lester Hayman (first recipient, also see Chapters 3, 7, 8, 10 and Appendix F), Gordon A. Bergy (sixth recipient, also see Chapters 1, 5, 7, 8, 10 and Appendix F), Frederick L. Geiler (12th recipient, also see Chapter 8 and Appendix F), Albert F. Wojcik (17th recipient, also see Chapter 8 and Appendix F) and Douglas D. Glover (20th recipient, also see Chapter 5 and Appendix F).

The annual Bowl of Hygeia Award is named for the mythological Greek goddess of health who is the source of the word "hygiene." Hygeia and her sister Panacea were daughters of Asclepios, the god of healing. The Award, for many years bestowed by the A. H. Robins company, is now sponsored by Wyeth-Ayerst Laboratories. The Bowl of Hygeia Award's purpose is to recognize an outstanding record of community service that reflects well on the profession. Each state presents this award, as well as the District of Columbia, Puerto Rico, and ten Canadian provinces.

The qualifications for the Bowl of Hygeia Award in West Virginia include the following requirements:

1. Member of WVPA and a resident of West Virginia
2. Must be a West Virginia licensed pharmacist
3. Must be living. Awards are not presented posthumously
4. Must not be a previous recipient of the award

5. Not currently serving, nor has served within the immediate past 2 years, as an officer of WVPA in other than an ex-officio capacity on its awards committee

6. Must have compiled an outstanding record of community service, which apart from his or her specific identification as a pharmacist reflects well on the profession

With perhaps the exception of medicine, pharmacy has enjoyed an association with community service longer than any other profession. This relationship probably also antedates recorded history. As a term, "community service" has a broad spectrum of definitions that tend to be an advantage rather than a detriment in selecting an award recipient. The only constant related to community service is the word "uncompensated." Although records from the Award's early selection process no longer exist, published reports in *The West Virginia Pharmacist* regarding Bowl of Hygeia awardees suggest that prior to 1980, activities benefiting the community as a whole received the greatest consideration.

To qualify for the Bowl of Hygeia Award, the recipient must have an exemplary service record. One such pharmacist was Miss Ann Dinardi, the 1963 Bowl of Hygeia recipient (also see Chapter 12). Ann was a leader who not only enhanced the quality of life in her community, but also impacted the lives of many individuals. [2]

Joseph G. Stevens received the Bowl of Hygeia in 1967 for his many years of work in the U.S. Coast Guard Auxiliary in the Cabell County, West Virginia area. Ironically, West Virginia is a landlocked state noted for its trout streams and rivers rather than oceans or seas, where one would least expect the United States Coast Guard to have a presence. Joe was in the Auxiliary for many years, serving as Commander of Flotilla 18-4. He supported the Coast Guard's work in responding to disasters in the shipping lanes of the Ohio River that include the dam and locks at Huntington. [3] Joe is retired and resides in Clearwater, Florida.

Although Rabbi Isadore "Izzy" R. Wein had an extensive resume of community service, his work with the youth of Beckley was paramount in his selection for the 1969 Bowl of Hygeia Award. A native of Harrison, New Jersey, Rabbi Wein was a son of Austrian immigrants and a 1934 graduate of Rutgers University College of Pharmacy. Izzy then attended New York University where, in 1936, he received a Bachelor of Science degree in chemistry, followed by a degree from the New Jersey Rabbinical Seminary.

Rabbi Wein met his future wife, Jeanette Abrams, on a blind date in New York. By coincidence, the date was on both Saint Patrick's Day and Palm Sunday; these two holidays fall on the same day only once in 300 years. Since Jeanette was a West Virginian, they initially had a long distance courtship. However, Izzy later moved to West Virginia to marry Jeanette and remained in Raleigh County for many years.

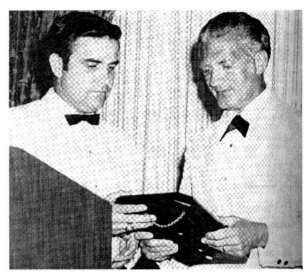

Isadore Wein (right) Receiving the 1969 Bowl of Hygeia Award

Izzy accepted a pharmacist's position at Raleigh General Hospital in Beckley and soon was actively involved with the community. Izzy found his nitch working with teenage boys; he kept them busy constructing tennis courts and then provided the teens with free tennis lessons. Izzy Wein also founded the local Woodlawn Boy's Club whose membership at one time included 35 local youngsters.[4] As Rabbi, Wein volunteered as chaplain for Jewish residents at the Beckley Veterans Administration Hospital, and he provided rabbinical services at the federal prison for women in Alderson, West Virginia.[4] Izzy was considered the most active man in Raleigh County: for 12 years he served as president of the Raleigh County branch of the American Cancer Society, was director of the Home Health Agency, and was active in the Community Concert Association. Izzy also served on the advisory council of the Appalachian Regional Hospital and for six years was chairman of the county Human Rights Commission. Rabbi Wein died in Greensboro, North Carolina, on February 11, 2000.

Seven Bowl of Hygeia Award recipients served as mayors of their West Virginia hometowns, with municipal government service contributing to their award selection. These individuals are William Sidney Coleman of Lewisburg (1966), Bill Plyburn of Barboursville (1971), Carl Furbee, Jr. of Bridgeport (1974), John Rice of Shinnston (1979), Sam Kapourales of Williamson (1982), George Karos of Martinsburg (1986), and Lydia Main of

Masontown (2002). The community service provided by these pharmacist-mayors is discussed in Chapter 3.

Wilbur Ernest Turner, the 1988 Bowl of Hygeia recipient, distinguished himself as a provider of services for the medically underserved individuals of the Huntington, West Virginia, area. Ernest was a director of Ebenezer Medical Outreach, a freestanding program for the medically underserved that is extant today. The mission of Ebenezer was to provide access to free, comprehensive health care, preventive care, and pharmaceuticals to the underserved residents of Huntington and surrounding areas. Ebenezer was guided by a system of beliefs recognizing health care as a basic right to which all are entitled. Ernest also worked with the Stella Fuller Settlement in Huntington that provides support for utilities, medicines, food and clothing to the economically disadvantaged, handicapped and elderly without charge regardless of national origin or race.[5] Ernest further served as president and provided more than 20 years of service to the West Huntington Kiwanis Club, and he chaired its fundraising committees to help the less fortunate in the Huntington-East area.[6]

Charles Vinton Selby, Jr., the 1992 Bowl of Hygeia Award recipient, is both a hospital and a community pharmacist. After graduating from the WVU School of Pharmacy, Charles served for two years as a line officer in the U.S. Navy. After completing his tour of service, he managed two independent community pharmacies in north central West Virginia before being selected pharmacist in charge of the Appalachian Regional Hospital in Beckley, West Virginia. Most recently, Charles served as director of pharmacy of a federally funded health care facility for low-income patients and as pharmacist/pharmacy computer specialist at the Veterans Administration Medical Center in Beckley. Volunteer service with the WVPA includes chairing the time-consuming third party Drug Utilization Review Committee and serving as treasurer and president of the Association.[7]

Donley W. Hutson was selected to receive the 1994 Bowl of Hygeia Award for the volunteer service he provided to county government, a municipal health clinic, and his church. Don is also justly proud of his 20 years of service on the Nutter Fort police Civil Service Commission. He served several times in each of three commission offices over two decades, as chairman, vice chairman, and recording secretary. For 16 years, he provided pharmacy services at the free Health Access Clinic in Clarksburg that provides care for individuals who are unable to afford private medical care but are not eligible for Medicaid. Don saves the clinic thousands of dollars annually by obtaining their drugs from a manufacturer with West Virginia ties. He serves on the clinic's Board of Directors and thoroughly enjoys his work there, adding he "works the clinic" about as much as he does his "real job." Additionally, Don is active in his church and has served as deacon, moderator, Sunday school teacher and as a member of the Budget and Finance Committee.

Carol Hudachek, the 2000 Bowl of Hygeia Award recipient, was a high school science teacher and assistant principal who later became a hospital pharmacist. Carol tells of the time when Dr. Carl Malanga, an emeritus professor at the WVU School of Pharmacy (see Chapter 8), came to the high school where she taught to speak to the students about pharmacy as a career. Later turning to her, Carl inquired why Carol herself hadn't considered a career in pharmacy. With much introspection as a result of that encounter, Carol enrolled in pharmacy school at West Virginia University with some of her former high school students who were now classmates. Blessed with a natural ability to communicate, Carol has employed this talent to develop a local broadcasting career in which she discusses appropriate medication use with the lay public.[8]

Lora Lewellyn Good, the 2003 Bowl of Hygeia recipient, has distinguished herself as a founder of the Queen for a Day/Heroes (QFAD) chapter in West Virginia. QFAD is a national non-profit organization dedicated to boosting the self-confidence of children with cancer. A fireman or policeman assists with their events, serving as an exemplar of the courage necessary to combat cancer or to fight fire and crime. Events are held throughout the year and are tailor-made to achieve the desires of each child participant. Lora also sponsors a float in the Stern Wheel Regatta parade as well as a dinner to lift the spirits and to honor children who have survived cancer.[9]

Nine pharmacists have received both the Dr. James H. Beal and the Bowl of Hygeia Awards. They include some truly remarkable individuals, one of whom was Jack E. Fruth, a native of Point Pleasant, West Virginia. Through his many years of pharmacy practice, Jack distinguished himself as an entrepreneur, businessman, community activist, and philanthropist. According to *Drug Store News,* in 2005 the Fruth chain was the 23rd largest retail pharmacy chain in the nation.[10] As of 2006, his chain of 22 pharmacies extended from Winfield, West Virginia, to Belpre, Ohio, and provided employment to over 500 people. Jack was a businessman who knew his customers personally and stressed customer service. He would go out of his way to provide the products his customers wanted, often with home delivery rather than necessitate a second trip by the customer to the pharmacy. After a warehouse fire disrupted the efficiency of his stores' operations, employees delivered merchandise from store to store by their own automobile as a temporary solution. Employer loyalty was paramount to his business plan: he would go to great lengths to avoid laying off an employee.[10] College scholarships, based on financial need and funded by Fruth Pharmacy, provided many Mason County youths an opportunity they would not otherwise have had to obtain a college education.[10] Jack was also a staunch promoter of

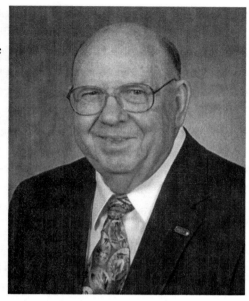

Jack Fruth - 1977 Bowl of Hygeia Award Recipient

business for Mason County, West Virginia, and lobbied for improvements of Mason County roads to enhance the business climate.[11] He was a director of a facility providing care for mentally handicapped youth. Jack was a trustee of Rio Grande (Ohio) University (across the state line from Point Pleasant, West Virginia) and, in 1986, the University recognized Jack for his service to Mason County by awarding him an Honorary Master of Public Service degree.[12] In 1993, Jack's *alma mater,* The Ohio State University College of Pharmacy, conferred upon him The Ohio State University Distinguished Alumnus Award.[13] West Virginia also recognized her native son. The WVPA awarded Fruth the Bowl of Hygeia Award in 1977 and the Dr. James H. Beal Award in 1995, and in 1999 Republican Governor Cecil Underwood presented Jack with the West Virginia Entrepreneur of the Year Lifetime Achievement Award.[13, 14] In recognition of Jack's work during his administration in early 2005, Democrat Governor Bob Wise designated U.S. Route 35 in Mason County the Fruth-Lanham Highway. Twenty days before Fruth's death on July 19, 2005, Jack met with current Governor Joe Manchin who committed himself to upgrade Route 35 to a four-lane structure, with construction to begin in four years.[15, 16]

West Virginia State Senator Charles C. Lanham wrote the following about Fruth shortly after Jack's death, "A most difficult challenge is to translate into words a proper description of Jack's leadership and vision. Jack could have a tremendous calming effect on any discussion regardless of the emotions involved. [Jack is] best described by the statement [that he] always got his brain in gear before he got his mouth in motion. Jack was a tremendous community leader." [17]

Thomas E. Menighan, the 1984 Bowl of Hygeia and the 1999 Beal Honor Award recipient, is another entrepreneur, pharmaceutical consultant, and a long-term activist with the American Pharmaceutical Association (also see Chapters 9, 10, and Appendices D, E).[18] Tom writes the following about his receipt of the Bowl of Hygeia award, "It was (and is to this day) one of the biggest honors of my life. At that time I was on the board of the West Virginia Division of the American Cancer Society (with Cecil Underwood) and served as president of the Cabell County unit." Tom was also involved in many other activities most of which were undertaken to promote West Virginia pharmacists rather than Tom's interests. Tom's selection as a Bowl of Hygeia recipient was in recognition of his extensive work and countless successes in the area of community service.[10]

David Stephen Crawford, the 1983 Dr. James Hartley Beal Award recipient, distinguished himself as a leader in the profession who served as president of three major pharmacy organizations, the West Virginia Pharmacists Association, American Pharmaceutical Association (and chairman of its Board of Trustees), and American Society of Hospital Pharmacists, now the American Society of Health-System Pharmacists (also see Chapters 6 and 9). He was a member of the West Virginia Health Advisory Committee and the Statewide Health Coordinating Council. Steve attracted national attention to West Virginia by creating a solution for a widespread problem, the paucity of pharmacists in small rural hospitals. Hospital administrators in rural communities often circumvent hiring pharmacists by utilizing nurses to dispense medications to reduce expenses, and they then justify the omission on an economic basis. Steve formed a corporation to provide pharmaceutical services for such hospitals. His corporate pharmacists were "circuit riders" who satisfied the individual needs of many such institutions for an affordable expense. As a result of his contribution to the public welfare of central West Virginia, Steve was selected the 1987 Bowl of Hygeia recipient by the WVPA. National recognition followed when Steve was selected as the first recipient of the APhA Practice Excellence Award, administered through the APhA Academy of Pharmacy Practice and Management.[19] Unfortunately, Steve died unexpectedly in early 2007.

Sandra Elizabeth Justice, the 1991 Bowl of Hygeia and the 1997 Dr. James H. Beal Award recipient, has established herself as a leader in the profession (also see Chapters 10, 12 and Appendices E, F). She served as a member of the West Virginia Board of Pharmacy, a compounding pharmacist, and a pharmaceutical consultant. Sandra was selected to receive the Bowl of Hygeia Award because of her contributions to pharmacy practice in West Virginia.[20] She served as a member of the West Virginia Medicaid Retro Drug Utilization Committee and as a private consultant for drug utilization program management and continuing education program development.[20] Sandra currently co-owns (with her husband) a compounding pharmacy in Indianapolis, but retains her strong ties to WVU as a member of the School of Pharmacy's Board of Advisors.

Thomas Lee Carson is the only honoree to have received both the Bowl of Hygeia and the Beal Award in the same year, 1993. Tom and his brother also practiced their entire 29-year career in a single pharmacy in Montgomery, West Virginia. Tom further served his community as director of the Merchants National Bank, director of the Upper Kanawha Valley Chamber of Commerce, and as director of the Upper Kanawha Valley Economic Development Association.

The Distinguished Young Pharmacist Award and the Innovative Pharmacy Practice Award are more recent honors given by WVPA. These award recipients are found in Appendix F. It is interesting to note that three of the Distinguished Young Pharmacist Award winners, Reed, Hudachek, and Lewellyn, later became Bowl of Hygeia recipients. Each of the other awardees has also distinguished himself or herself in their profession or community. These award recipients exemplify the generally understated and often unrecognized caring, service-oriented nature of pharmacists.

Chapter Twelve

Women as Leaders
in the Profession

A century has passed since Willa Hood Strickler joined the West Virginia Pharmaceutical Association in 1907 as its first female member. However, the gender shift that would eventually occur was gradual, with women showing little interest in pharmacy as a profession for several decades. Of the 84 graduates from the Department of Pharmacy of the WVU College of Medicine from 1917 to 1930, only nine (10.7 %) were female. Of those, one received a four-year bachelor of science (B.S.) degree, four elected to obtain the three-year pharmaceutical chemist (Ph.C.) degree, and four earned a two-year pharmaceutical graduate (Ph.G.) degree that was the most popular degree with men.[a] Not only did women perform as well as their male counterparts in the classroom, they favored the more academically challenging and rigorous education programs. Thus, the paucity of women in the profession in the early years of the 20th century represented a matter of choice rather than a lack of ability.

Of the various U.S. professional schools of that era, more women graduated from schools of pharmacy where they were more likely to be accepted for admission compared to other professional schools such as medicine, dentistry or law. This was also the case in West Virginia. During the decade of the 1930s, seven of 62 pharmacy graduates (11.3 %) were female, compared to 19 of the 399 medical graduates (4.7%) and eight of the 153 law graduates (5.2%). However, pharmacy was still a man's profession at that time.

Although their numbers were relatively small, female pharmacists who graduated between 1920 and 1950 gradually began to exert leadership in the profession. Alice Collins Bennett of Fairmont (Marion County), West

---

[a] *Cecelia Kranaskas Kay in 1928 received a bachelor's degree from the Department of Pharmacy, one of only two such degrees granted from 1917 to 1930.*

Virginia was an early example. Born December 17, 1900, Alice was a 1923 graduate of the WVU Department of Pharmacy. Alice opened her own pharmacy on Fairmont's east side, the only pharmacy on that side of town. Alice was one of the early (if not the first) female pharmacy owners in West Virginia and was also president of the Marion County Pharmaceutical Association. Pharmacy ownership was a bold undertaking for a woman of that era. Without hesitation, Alice exerted pharmacy leadership as no West Virginia woman had dared to do before.

When Alice sold her pharmacy to Dan Rider in 1966, which he continues to own to this day, she relinquished a leadership role she had held for 43 years. But Alice didn't retire with the sale of her pharmacy; she continued to practice with Dan for another decade. Dan tells of his early association with Alice Bennett, for whom he interned for a year before taking the licensing examination. Alice had offered to hire Dan when he became licensed. The day he walked into the pharmacy after passing the board examination, Alice greeted him with, "OK, there it is," and left the pharmacy. From that day on, Alice assumed the role of an employee with Dan as the boss. It was time for her to slow down but she was determined not to quit. Dan operated the drug store as if it was his pharmacy without interference from Alice. A year later when Dan planned to take a position with a pharmacy in Parkersburg, Alice asked him to buy her store. Since Dan lacked sufficient money for such a purchase, Alice offered to co-sign a note for a loan. However, they were unsuccessful in negotiating a loan locally, with one banker suggesting that Fairmont had too many pharmacies. Unperturbed, Alice took Dan to Clarksburg where Lane Exley, president of Clarksburg Drug Company, arranged a loan there. Once the purchase of Bennett Pharmacy was accomplished, Alice stayed with Dan to help him get established in the community. "She taught me a lot of things; she taught me how to relate to people and the business just took off from there," Dan says. "She worked for practically nothing to get me started," he added. Alice Bennett retired in 1976 and died March 22, 1995, at the age of 94.[1]

Ann Dinardi, a 1931 graduate of the WVU Department of Pharmacy, was another woman who owned her own pharmacy and was known for her early leadership role in pharmacy practice. Born on September 8, 1906, Ann grew up in a family of eleven children in Mount Union, Pennsylvania, a rural community located near Harrisburg. After graduating from high school, Ann moved to Morgantown to baby-sit for her older sister Julia's children. Julia was married to a successful Morgantown businessman, Sam Chico, a dairy owner who wanted Ann to attend college. Ann lacked confidence in her intellectual ability and told Sam she was "'too dumb" to succeed. Nonetheless, he convinced Ann that her ability was certainly sufficient to successfully complete at least a college course and offered to pay her expenses.[2] Ann not only completed a course, she enrolled in the West Virginia University College of Pharmacy pharmaceutical chemist program in 1928, a much more rigorous program than the two-year pharmaceutical graduate curriculum that most aspiring pharmacists completed those days.

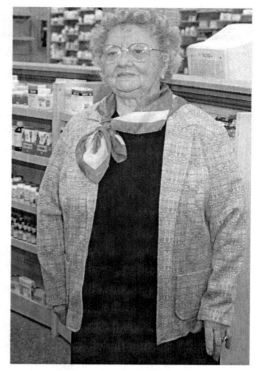

Ann Dinardi (1980)

As a freshman, Ann wished to join a sorority but was not allowed to rush due to her Italian heritage; Italians were considered "undesirable" by fraternal organizations in the 1920s. Her response to rejection by campus Greeks was typical of Ann: she founded her own sorority, Beta Iota, with membership limited to women of Italian heritage.[2] Receiving her Ph.C. degree in 1931, Ann was the eighth woman to graduate from the fledgling pharmacy school and the first alumnus of Italian heritage.[2]

From 1931 to 1947, Ann was employed as a staff pharmacist at a local chain pharmacy. She then joined pharmacist Mary Angotti, also a WVU College of Pharmacy graduate, to purchase Moore and Parriot Drug Store in downtown Morgantown to start their own practice, a partnership that endured for 35 years. They did not rename the newly purchased pharmacy to take advantage of their Italian names,[2] despite the strategic influence this may have had on the substantial Italian population then residing in Morgantown and the surrounding area.

These two young pharmacists were not shrinking violets; they were both active in the local business community. Ann joined the Quota Club and she became active in the Business and Professional Woman's Club and the Catholic Daughters. It didn't take long for Ann's attributes to be recognized by the municipal and university communities. She was named district chairman of the National Federation of Independent Business, a member of the Small Business Advisory Council for West Virginia's Region III, and a council member of Morgantown's Downtown Action Committee.[3]

Ever loyal to her university, Ann became housemother for the Alpha Phi Delta fraternity, known as the "Italian" fraternity, then active on the WVU campus. In 1939, Ann's sister Julia and her husband bought a house on Beechurst Avenue near the Old Field House, now Stansbury Hall, for Ann to live in. Three years later they gave Ann the deed.[3] This simple, thoughtful gesture would turn out to affect not only the rest of Ann's life but the lives of many other individuals.

A sports enthusiast of football and basketball in particular, Ann identified a need not previously addressed by the University community: a means by which a student athlete, unable to afford a college education, could receive help within the legal and ethical constraints of the day to attend West Virginia University. Ann's brother, Sy Dinardi, recalls Ann making the house at 65 Beechurst Avenue[b] available to these student athletes even though it was quite small.[4] During the winter months she provided rooms for three or four students which increased to five or six students in the summer months because they had nowhere else to stay.[4] Initially Ann took in football players. These students were like family to Ann; she insisted they complete their education, unlike many college football programs of that era. Star players or not, they were all treated alike. In time, the student mix shifted from football to basketball.

Ann gave nationally known athletes Jerry West and Rod Hundley (both of whom also stayed with Ann) "hell" when they felt sorry for themselves, telling them if they didn't want an education they could leave her home. Ann was also a disciplinarian, according to Buddy Quertinmont, a former basketball player. "On the first day of class, Ann made a list of everyone's class schedule with the names of their professors. She personally called each professor requesting that she be notified if one of us missed a class. If Ann found that a student-athlete was missing class, she would get upset. When Ann became exasperated with the basketball players, she was prone to use rather salty language. After an episode of choice epithets, Ann would often say, 'Well, I will have to go to church and confess for that.'" [5] Ann's method of "persuasion" worked; only one of the estimated 30 basketball players who stayed with Ann did not graduate from the University, an admirable

---

[b] *The house was demolished in 2008.*

achievement. Later in life, a number of these players became successful coaches, including Gale Catlett at West Virginia University and others, such as Willie Akers, as high school coaches.

Ann charged the student-athletes $7.00 a week rent, provided they had the funds. In return, Ann stocked the refrigerator with meat.[4] Buddy Quertinmont also tells about walking up the street to her pharmacy to visit: "When you left the pharmacy you had to leave with a package or she would be upset with you. She would give us toothpaste, soap and after-shave lotion...she was such a giving person, and she was like that all her life." [5]

Ann Dinardi's philanthropy also transcended to her pharmacy. One day a young man nervously handed Ann a prescription to be filled; he had a new sick baby at home. Ann filled the prescription and handed the medication to the young father, who inquired about its cost. When told the price of the prescription, he broke down. With tears streaming down his cheeks he looked at Ann and said, "Why didn't somebody tell me getting married and having babies was going to cost so much?" Appreciating the young man's dilemma, Ann asked how much money he had. When he replied "two dollars," Ann accepted one dollar, then gave him back fifty cents on the agreement he would pay the balance of the prescription price in twenty-five cent increments as his financial circumstances permitted. It took nearly a year for the young man to complete the payments, but when he did Ann refunded his money in full.[6]

Always active in the WVU School of Pharmacy Alumni Association, Ann Dinardi was elected secretary-treasurer of the Association in 1941. Along with alumni Joe Nemeth and Ed Rockis, she did much of the "behind the scenes" preparation for the Annual Pharmacy Alumni Banquet each year. Ann's hard work as an officer of the Association was recognized by the membership and did not go unappreciated. She was reelected secretary-treasurer year after year, essentially by acclimation, as no one would oppose her for re-election. In 2000, she announced she would not stand for re-election. Ann had given more of her time and effort than ever expected, serving as an officer of the Association over an unprecedented span of 59 years.

A little known fact about Ann Dinardi was her scholarship philanthropy that antedates the organized University scholarship program. Ann made gifts directly to students in need of financial assistance. She paved the way for many students, not necessarily limited to pharmacy students or student athletes, to attend the University. For others, in lieu of financial help she arranged part-time jobs. No record exists of the number of students who benefited from Ann's generosity over the years.

A very modest woman, Ann Dinardi was never one to seek public recognition for her deeds. Nonetheless, she has been honored eight times by her *alma mater* and state professional organizations. The School of Pharmacy recognized her on three occasions, with the Outstanding Service Award in 1952 and 1969 and the Outstanding Alumnus Award in 1957. In 1963, the WVPA recognized her philanthropy by awarding her the Bowl of Hygeia Award. In 1997, the University conferred upon her its highest award, the Order of Vandalia, the only pharmacist to be so honored. In 1989, she was selected as the Homecoming parade marshal and was named "Mountaineer Mother" in recognition of all the years she served as "Mother" to some very famous student athletes. Additionally, Ann has been honored through two scholarships endowed in her name: the Ann Dinardi Basketball Scholarship endowment in 1996, and the Jerry and Karen West and Ann Dinardi Basketball Scholarship in 2004. These are fitting legacies to a woman who had done so much for students and who will always be remembered by her many friends and colleagues in the athletic and pharmacy fields. When Ann Dinardi passed away in October 2003, her funeral was attended by many of the athletes she nurtured over the years.

A published study from the Philadelphia College of Pharmacy in the early 1940s confirmed the West Virginia data of two decades earlier, that the academic performance of female students equaled that of their male counterparts. Yet, only 4% of pharmacists practicing in the Philadelphia area at that time were female. Women were proving they could successfully complete a professional pharmacy program; now, it was a matter of getting more to apply for admission. With the end of the depression, male enrollment in the WVU College of Pharmacy escalated while that of women did not change. War served as the impetus for the needed change. With the entry of the United States into World War II, military requirements virtually eliminated higher education's male applicant pool. Following the Japanese attack on Pearl Harbor and Germany's declaration of war on the United States in December 1941, male graduation rates initially rose and then fell as men left school to enter the armed services (Table 1). In order to remain open during the war years, the nations' pharmacy schools undertook recruitment programs for female students. Although female enrollment increased during the war, the graduation rates for women were only modestly changed by the end of that decade. By the end of the war, the nation was experiencing a pharmacist shortage that could not be solely addressed by military demobilization. U.S. pharmacy schools responded to this need by increasing class sizes, adding night and Saturday classes and offering more than one entry class a year. As a result, female enrollment in pharmacy schools gradually increased.

As the 1940s drew to a close, females comprised 20.6% of pharmacy graduates compared to 13.8% in the immediate pre-war years.[c] To recruit more women, WVU pharmacy school Dean J. Lester Hayman actively promoted pharmacy as the ideal profession for a woman. As a result of his efforts and those of other administrators and faculty, female enrollment in pharmacy school from 1950 to 1980 escalated, and the percentage of women graduates in the 1970s doubled that of the 1950s. As the end of the 20th century approached, the profession underwent dramatic changes. No longer was the "corner drug store" open 14 hours a day from 8 AM to 10 PM. Hospital pharmacy was no longer relegated to a back corner of the basement. Decentralized hospital pharmacy became a reality, and other venues for a pharmacist to advance in his or her professional career became numerous. Pharmacists entered the pharmaceutical industry as pharmacologists, researchers, sales representatives and information specialists. Each of these changes made the profession more attractive to women.

In November 2006, the four schools of the West Virginia University Health Sciences Center (HSC) honored women for their commitment and accomplishments in their respective professions. The Executive Committee of the School of Pharmacy, with input from faculty, selected 16 honorees that met the HSC's criteria for women whose careers had achieved both state and national recognition. Of these outstanding woman leaders, three were academicians, eight were community pharmacists, two were hospital pharmacists, and one each was a highly successful entrepreneur, a state government insurance program administrator, and an executive of the American Pharmacists Association. Dr. Marie Abate is one of the academicians the Executive Committee selected.

Dr. Abate joined the faculty of the WVU School of Pharmacy in 1981. She was the only woman on the School of Pharmacy's faculty at the time. Born in Detroit, Michigan, Marie grew up in the suburb of East Detroit now called Eastpointe. A graduate of the University of Michigan, she received a Bachelor of Science degree in pharmacy in 1979 and a Doctor of Pharmacy

---

[c] *Specific WVU enrollment data are not available. Graduate data were determined by averaging the number of graduates in the last three years of each respective decade.*

degree in 1981, graduating at the top of her class in both programs. As an undergraduate student, Marie was very introverted and rarely spoke out during class. She still remembers one of the University of Michigan College of Pharmacy faculty members telling her during an interview for a spot in the Doctor of Pharmacy degree program that they weren't sure whether they should accept her because she was too quiet.

Fate played a prominent role in Dr. Abate's appointment as a WVU faculty member. Her primary interest area at that time was adult internal medicine. A few months prior to graduation, Marie participated in the personnel placement service at the American Society of Hospital Pharmacists' Midyear Clinical Meeting and saw an ad for an available faculty position at the WVU School of Pharmacy. The ad sought an individual with interest in adult internal medicine who would serve as vice-chair of the School's Charleston Division. However, Marie misread the ad and thought that two positions were available, one for an adult internal medicine faculty member, of some interest to her, and a second for a vice-chair. She arranged an interview with the chair of the WVU Department of Clinical Pharmacy at that time and was completely caught off guard by his first question, "So why are you interested in the vice-chair position at WVU?" Having not yet graduated, with no administrative experience, Marie quickly apologized for her misunderstanding of the position. Although she followed through on formally applying for the vice-chair position, she understandably was not hired for it.[7] However, in March 1981, she was invited to formally interview for a faculty position in internal medicine/drug information in Morgantown. Marie ultimately accepted the position of Assistant Professor of Clinical Pharmacy beginning July 1981, on the condition that she would be able to shift into a new internal medicine only position when it became available the following year. By the time the medicine position became available, Marie enjoyed her practice as a drug information specialist. Marie often tells pharmacy students this story as an illustration of why they need to keep an open mind about different specialty areas; sometimes you end up in places that you never initially dreamed you would. When Marie first moved to West Virginia, her mother gave her as a gift a clock carved of wood shaped like the state of West Virginia and said, "This will be a nice memento for when you leave here." Twenty-seven years later, the clock still works and Marie has it in her home in Morgantown.[7]

Marie Abate is nationally recognized and respected for her expertise in the area of drug information. She has served as director of the statewide West Virginia Center for Drug and Health Information (WV CDHI), a service for health care professionals, for the past 20 years. During that time, the Center has expanded its services to include outreach to patients through the provision of high quality Internet-based health information. Dr. Abate has served as an investigator on over 20 funded research and educational projects totaling almost $1.5 million. With colleagues, she developed an innovative computer education program to teach students how to interpret and assess medical literature that has been used at WVU for 15 years as well as at a number of other schools of pharmacy. This work received an Innovations in Teaching Award from the American Association of Colleges of Pharmacy. She is currently collaborating with the West Virginia Office of the Chief Medical Examiner in developing a forensic drug information web site and database. Dr. Abate has served as director of assessment for the School where she has helped to develop the School's learning outcomes assessment plan. Marie has also conducted faculty development seminars and workshops about assessment within the School, Health Sciences Center (HSC), and nationally at workshops sponsored by the American Association of Colleges of Pharmacy.[7]

Dr. Virginia (Ginger) Scott, like Dr. Abate, is another academician who is recognized for her teaching, research, and leadership in the profession. Born in Somerset, Kentucky, Ginger received a Bachelor of Science in pharmacy degree from the University of Kentucky in 1972 and a Master of Science in pharmacy administration degree from Purdue University in 1991. With research in pharmaceutical economics, she earned a Ph.D. degree in social and administrative pharmacy from the University of Minnesota in 1996. Ginger began pharmacy practice as a community pharmacist in Kentucky and practiced for 22 years in both community and hospital settings. Not only was she the first woman to serve as president of the Kentucky Pharmacists Association, she has also served as president of the Kentucky Society of Health-System Pharmacists.[8] Ginger joined the WVU School of Pharmacy faculty in 1994 and has served as director of continuing education (CE) for the last 10 years. Under her leadership, the School's CE programming and impact have grown dramatically. The School is now the largest provider of CE in West Virginia. Her vision for the program has been to offer not only traditional CE programming, but also training to enhance pharmacy practitioners' ability to provide medication therapy management services that optimize patient outcomes and improve quality of life.

Dr. Scott is nationally known for her expertise in CE. Currently, she serves as a member of the CE Advisory Committee for the *Annals of Pharmacotherapy* and as past-chair of the Continuing Pharmacy Education section. Ginger also serves as chair of the Academic Sections Coordinating Committee and member of the Board of Directors of the American Association of Colleges of Pharmacy (AACP). Her research interest focuses on continuing professional development of pharmacists and health care quality improvement.[8]

Elizabeth Jane Scharman is the third female academician selected for recognition for her leadership in the profession of pharmacy. Born in Camp LeJeaune, North Carolina (where her naval medical officer father was stationed), and reared in Utah, Elizabeth worked as a research technician in biochemistry at the University of Utah Medical Center while still attending high school. Her work gave her an opportunity to think about her future career. Although she loved science, she found she did not want to work in a laboratory. Elizabeth started attending the University of Utah the summer before her senior year in high school and continued to attend part-time during her senior year. As a pre-med major, she took an elective course called "Common Medicines" to learn how medications worked. A guest lecturer in that class was the director of the Utah Poison Center and a dynamic speaker. Elizabeth left the class thinking, "I love the topic of clinical toxicology and would love to do what he does." The speaker was a pharmacist; therefore, she reasoned, "in order to do what he does I need to be a pharmacist." She changed her major the next day. Pharmacy, she concluded, combined her love of medicine and science so she felt it was a good fit. "At the time, I had no idea what pharmacy was all about or what pharmacists did. I had never stepped foot in a pharmacy. I just knew that I wanted to do what the director did. I had always wanted to attend school out of state, so it was logical to move when it was time to enroll in pharmacy school." [9]

After graduation from Murray High School in 1981, Elizabeth enrolled in the pre-pharmacy program at the University of Utah. In June 1983, she transferred to Butler University in Indianapolis, Indiana, where she received a Bachelor of Science degree in pharmacy in 1986. A position was available in Louisiana for a full-time poison information specialist at the Louisiana Poison Center in Shreveport, where she worked for a year along with relief work as a community pharmacist. Elizabeth loved her job in Louisiana, where she gained a wealth of experience. However, she hated the humidity and cajun food, so she accepted a position as a full-time hospital pharmacist and part-time poison information specialist at the Central Virginia Poison Center in Richmond,

Virginia. Enrolling in the Virginia Commonwealth University (Medical College of Virginia) Pharm.D. program in August 1989, she graduated with honors and received her degree in 1991. That year was a momentous year for Elizabeth: she was inducted into the Rho Chi honor society and received the Upjohn Research Award and the Clinical Pharmacy Practice award. Elizabeth subsequently completed a clinical toxicology fellowship at the Pittsburgh Poison Center/University of Pittsburgh and was named director of the West Virginia Poison Center in Charleston on July 1, 1992. [9]

When she accepted the Poison Center director position, Elizabeth's education objectives had been achieved. In the process, she had moved around much of the United States and wanted to settle down. However, was West Virginia the state for her? Experience told her she preferred life in a city and certainly did not want to live in a rural locale. But she had no money and was tired of moving. "I can do anything for three years," she told herself. Fifteen years have now passed; she is still in Charleston, is married to a native West Virginian and is the mother of two small children. Elizabeth has been successful in her professional career, having served as president of the American Academy of Clinical Toxicology with recent reelection to a three-year term on its Board of Trustees. She is also past president of the American Board of Applied Toxicology. In July 2003, she was promoted to the rank of professor at West Virginia University School of Pharmacy.

The eight WVU Health Sciences Center honorees that are community pharmacists have very productive and diverse careers providing exemplary public service. Carol Hudachek is a typical example (also see Chapters 10, 11 and Appendices E, F). Although service has been the hallmark of her life, the profession of pharmacy was not her first career. Initially she was a teacher and a high school principal. Carol received a Bachelor of Arts degree in biology and a Master of Arts degree in education from West Virginia University in 1973 and 1977, respectively. According to Carol, "I got into teaching by accident. It was the middle of the school year and the school needed a science teacher. The principal, who knew my background, called and asked if I would be interested in teaching. At that time, I was working on my master's in microbiology and was a little frustrated with my research so I said, "Oh, sure. This may be a good opportunity for me. I'll take a semester or two off and then return to finish my master's." Carol ended up teaching in high school for 10 years and instead of a master's degree in biology, she received a master's degree in education. [10]

Communication is a common thread linking Carol's teaching and pharmacy careers. Carol has had a monthly "Ask the Pharmacist" radio program, with numerous broadcasts provided over the years to residents of the Wheeling-Steubenville area. On occasion, patients at Weirton Medical Center may recognize Carol's voice from her radio broadcasts. Carol's long-term commitment to pharmacy is extensive and includes service as president of the West Virginia Pharmacists Association (WVPA) as well as service to other professional organizations (see Appendix E). [10]

Another community pharmacist recognized by the WVU Health Sciences Center is Patricia Johnston (also see Chapter 10 and Appendix E). Patty is a 1977 graduate of the WVU School of Pharmacy, has served as president of the WVPA, and is the current past president of the WVU School of Pharmacy Alumni Association. Patty is president and owner of Colony Drug and Wellness Center, an independent community pharmacy in Beckley, West Virginia. Her pharmacy practice is focused on wellness screenings, compounding, disease management, and health and fitness services. Colony Drug also provides consultative services and medications for hospice needs in Raleigh County. Patty is a pioneer for change in the pharmacy profession. As a leader in championing collaborative pharmacy practice legislation in West Virginia, she has served as a member of the School of Pharmacy Collaborative Practice Committee and currently chairs the Task Force for Collaborative Practice. Such legislation, if passed, would allow pharmacists to enter into agreements with physicians to perform specified patient care services to optimize medication therapy. Patty is an adjunct faculty member of the School of Pharmacy and serves as a preceptor and role model for students. In 2001 and 2007, Patty was recognized as the School's Preceptor of the Year for excellence in experiential education. [11]

Reflecting back to her childhood, Patty recalls accompanying her father, pharmacist Harold Johnston (class of 1951), when he visited other pharmacies in Beckley. While her father chatted with a colleague, Patty and her sister "would scout the inventory and became experts as to which pharmacy [in Beckley] had the best selection of toys and candy." Her favorite pharmacy to visit was Colony Drug on Valley Drive. As Patty recalls, "That pharmacy had a humdinger of a soda fountain…the ice cream choices went beyond the pedestrian chocolate, vanilla, and strawberry to include an exotic and delicious flavor, black raspberry, unavailable elsewhere in my world." While young Patty spun on the red vinyl soda fountain stools at Colony Drug, she never dreamed that some day she and her father would own that very pharmacy. With the passing of her father in 1996, Patty had to decide whether to sell the pharmacy to a chain or keep it and carry on without him. Without much hesitation, she decided to keep it. Over the ensuing years, Colony Drug moved across the street and expanded and prospered, adding a fitness center. Currently, they are preparing to build an even larger facility to house their entire operation.

Sandra Justice, a daughter of a community pharmacist and a community pharmacist herself, has devoted as much of her professional life to organized pharmacy as she has to pharmacy practice. Born in Montgomery, West Virginia, Sandra graduated with a Bachelor of Pharmacy degree from the West Virginia University School of Pharmacy in 1978. However, pharmacy was not Sandy's first choice for a profession. Initially at college, she enrolled in a fashion merchandizing program and envisioned herself as a buyer for a big city department store. However, it didn't take long for Sandy to realize her true calling, and she applied for admission and was accepted into the School of Pharmacy. After graduation, Sandy returned to Montgomery to practice with her father, from whom she learned that satisfaction in life could best be derived from caring for people.[12]

Once established in practice, Sandra became active in the Upper Kanawha Valley Chamber of Commerce and was eventually elected president. Her leadership abilities having been recognized, Sandra was elected president of the West Virginia Pharmacists Association (also see Chapter 11), the first of her gender, just eight years after becoming a pharmacist. In 1990, she was elected president of the WVU School of Pharmacy Alumni Association and the following year Sandra received the School of Pharmacy Outstanding Service Award and was elected to Phi Lambda Sigma leadership honorary. She received the WVPA Presidents Award three times between 1989 and 1994. Service on the West Virginia Board of Pharmacy and a three-year term on the APhA Board of Trustees followed, and Sandra was named chair of the WVU School of Pharmacy Board of Advisors in 1995.[12]

Sandra's father died in 1996; thus, the impetus to commute 60 miles a day from Charleston to Montgomery no longer existed. At that time, Sandra was dating a pharmacy-owner in Indiana, and long distance courtships are difficult to sustain. Since Sandy shared his vision for pharmacy, she sold the pharmacy in Montgomery and moved to Indianapolis. Today, she and Charles operate Nora Apothecary in Indianapolis, Indiana, in a practice that focuses on prescription compounding.[12]

151

Susan Meredith is another community pharmacist honored by the HSC. A 1967 graduate of the WVU School of Pharmacy, she and her husband Ron (who died in 2007 after battling cancer), have owned and operated a pharmacy in Lumberport, West Virginia, since 1973. However, Susan's parents initially had other plans for their daughter. They wanted her to study music. At the age of five, Susan started piano lessons. But Susan had an idol who was also her role model, pharmacist Edward D. Tetrick (son of Arch Tetrick, see Chapters 3 and 10). When she was in the fourth grade, Susan told her parents she wanted to be a pharmacist like Ed. She persevered with piano lessons until her freshman year in high school, when her parents finally relinquished and let her discontinue the formal lessons. Susan was now on the path to the career she so desperately wanted. According to Susan, "In my class of 1967 at WVU, we had eight women (out of a class of 39). Ann Dinardi, class of 1931, was a huge influence on all of our lives. We were her girls. In Harrison County that year, only two women were practicing pharmacy. The biggest challenge I faced after graduation was to have the public accept me as a woman who was a registered pharmacist." However, Ed convinced some of the older, doubting patients that Susan was a well-trained pharmacist and before long, she was accepted. Susan practiced with Ed until his untimely death in 1970. After that, she and her husband purchased Lumberport Pharmacy. Susan adds, "My parents' desire for me to become a musician was somewhat fulfilled in that I still play the piano at home, the organ at my church, and also the alto saxophone in the Shinnston community band." Music appreciation, at least in the Meredith family, appears to be genetically determined. Their daughter, Betsy Elswick, is also a musician, having attended West Virginia Wesleyan College as a pre-pharmacy student where she was the pianist for the jazz ensemble and chapel choir and played clarinet in the concert band. Today, Betsy is a Clinical Assistant Professor of Pharmacy at WVU.

A community educator, Susan completed training in hyperlipidemia, diabetes, and immunization. She is a current participant in the Public Employees Insurance Agency's (PEIA) Face-to-Face Program in which she provides individual counseling to diabetes patients. A long time member of the WVU School of Pharmacy Alumni Association, Susan is a past co-president of the Association and currently serves as the Association's secretary. In 2006, Susan and her late husband Ron received the WVPA Community Service Award for their many community service activities, including providing drug abuse education programs for high school students and presentations on pharmacy as a career choice to middle school and high school students.[13]

Lydia Main is a community pharmacist/pharmacy owner in Masontown (Preston County), West Virginia. Lydia, whose maiden name was DeBoni, is rightfully proud of her Italian heritage. Her father immigrated to the United States in 1924 from Lentianara in the province of Belluno, a 90-minute drive from Venice. He settled in the community of Bretz, a mile from Masontown. In 1927, her father returned to Italy for a vacation where he met and married a woman seven years his junior. Her mother, eager to learn English, enrolled in the Masontown Elementary School where she spent two years becoming fluent in the language. Lydia, the eldest of two daughters, was born in September 1929. To help support the family, her mother ran a boarding house where she had 12 borders that either worked at the Bethlehem Steel facility in Bretz or the coke ovens in Richard, both small towns in Preston County.

Lydia Main's background was not indicative of her future successes. She has been a member of the State Board of Pharmacy for 20 years and currently serves as the Board's vice-president. She is a member of the National Association of Boards of Pharmacy and serves on the Task Force on Internet Pharmacy. She is the longest serving mayor in Masontown's history (see Chapter 3), having again been reelected in 2007. Lydia is a past president of the WVU School of Pharmacy Alumni Association.[14]

Karen Ellenbogen Reed is a community pharmacist who was selected for the HSC award for her professional leadership on the local, state, and national levels, for her teaching abilities, and for her community service. A 1980 graduate of the WVU School of Pharmacy, Karen was the only chain-store pharmacist selected for this honor, having previously been named by her employer as the 2003 K-mart Pharmacist of the Year. A past recipient of the West Virginia Pharmacists Association Distinguished Young Pharmacist Award, Karen has served the profession as president of the WVPA, president of the WVU School of Pharmacy Alumni Association, chair of the APhA-APPM Community and Ambulatory Section, and as a member of the Board of Trustees of the American Pharmacists Association. Karen's devotion to community service has been demonstrated by her effective leadership of the West Virginia Medicaid Drug Utilization Review Board and membership in many professional and civic organizations, for which she has been recognized with the Bowl of Hygeia Award. In the role of teacher, Karen stands out as a preceptor and role model for pharmacy students as an adjunct assistant professor for the School of Pharmacy, diabetes educator, consultant, and an American Pharmacists national spokesperson.

The focus of Karen's life since age five had been to become a pediatrician. However, in her senior year of high school, she fell in love with her future husband and her life changed. He wanted to be a pharmacist; today her husband is a medical sales representative for a major pharmaceutical company. Not wanting to be separated from him, Karen applied for admission to pharmacy school. Her decision to not become a pediatrician was confirmed during her pediatric rotation when Karen concluded that this specialty area was not her forte.[15]

Like many of her contemporaries, Barbara Dietz Smith left home for college unsure of what career path she wanted to travel. As a child, she played school and envisioned herself as a teacher. Preparing for this career, Glenville State College at Glenville, West Virginia, was selected due to its proximity to her home and teaching emphasis. In fact, Glenville State College had been chartered in 1872 as Glenville Normal School, a preparatory school for teachers. However, as the summer before her freshman year approached, Barbara had a change of heart and decided teaching was not what she wanted as a career. Living on a farm, she loved animals and small-animal veterinary medicine came to mind. However, her veterinarian talked her out of that option because of the competition for acceptance into veterinary school. Since Barbara knew she wanted to study something in the health-care field, she consulted her family pharmacist, Phil Keller, for advice. Phil was easy to talk with and suggested Barbara work with him in the pharmacy during a school break. He allowed her to observe what transpired in the prescription department. According to Barbara, she was "interested in the medicines – what the drugs were for – and how to give people advice and help them with their problems. The first day I worked for him I knew I wanted to be a pharmacist for the rest of my life." By the end of that day with Phil Keller, pharmacy was the career she wanted to pursue.

Despite making the decision years ago not to become a teacher, Barbara learned that a pharmacist is in fact a teacher. She is an adjunct assistant professor of pharmacy, a pharmacy field professor for the West Virginia Rural Health Education Partnership (WV RHEP) program, and a Certified Diabetes Educator. Barbara is an outstanding role model for her students during their community and ambulatory care rotations. With Barbara's intervention, diabetes awareness has increased in Spencer, West Virginia, where she has implemented the PEIA Face-to-Face diabetes program. In the year 2000, the West Virginia Pharmacists Association awarded Barbara its "Innovative Pharmacy Practice Award," and the following year she received the West Virginia Society of Health System Pharmacists' Roche Education Award for her commitment to health care education and excellence in teaching. The School of Pharmacy, in conjunction with Roche Laboratories, presented her with the 2002 Preceptor of the Year award. Barbara serves on the West Virginia Medicaid Retrospective Drug Utilization Review Committee and the West Virginia Board of Pharmacy Continuing Education Committee. [16]

Michele Vigneault McNeill is a successful entrepreneur who has played active roles in community pharmacy, hospital pharmacy, the pharmaceutical industry, and government. Born in Albany, New York, she spent her formative years in Charleston, West Virginia. Realizing she had an interest in the sciences early in her career, Michele first considered becoming a physician and enrolled in the pre-medicine program at West Virginia Wesleyan University. At Wesleyan, a friend talked her into transferring to WVU to enter its pharmacy program. As an undergraduate pharmacy student at WVU, Dr. Arthur Jacknowitz mentored Michele through the clinical pharmacy program and became a major influence in her life. Years later as an expression of her gratitude, Michele endowed the Arthur I. Jacknowitz Chair in Clinical Pharmacy, the School of Pharmacy's first endowed chair. Michele's clinical pharmacy career began at Thomas Jefferson University Hospital in Philadelphia where she managed a pharmacy satellite in the respiratory intensive care unit, followed by a short stay at the State University of New York as a drug information specialist. Moving to industry, Michele worked at Warner Lambert (later becoming a part of Pfizer), Hoffman La Roche, and Ciba Geigy (now Novartis), where she realized there was a need to bring community physicians, industry, and government together to provide early access to investigational drugs for serious and life-threatening diseases such as AIDS, hepatitis, and cancer. This became the vision for the company she founded, Kern McNeill International (KMI).

KMI was started in her home at the kitchen table. After 10 years growth, KMI had 150 employees worldwide and 50 million dollars in revenue when Michele decided to sell to a division of United Healthcare. Michele remained with the company for three additional years, during which the company continued to grow through mergers and acquisitions to over 1,300 employees in 20 countries, with $150 million in revenue. KMI pioneered the compassionate-use programs by which over 100,000 patients have been helped, most of whom were victims of HIV/AIDS or cancer. The new owners of the company have continued its compassionate-use program after Michele retired. In retirement, Michele continues her work with HIV/AIDS through the American Foundation for AIDS Research (AMFAR), which is dedicated to AIDS research, education for AIDS prevention, and public policy. Through her presidential appointment to the National Institutes of Health's Office of AIDS Research Advisory Council, she currently serves on the HIV/AIDS Therapeutic Working Group. With pride, Michele joins Frank Lilly (see Chapter 13) and Newell Stewart (see Appendix A) as the third WVU School of Pharmacy alumnus to receive a prestigious presidential appointment.[17] In 2005, Michele's *alma mater* WVU recognized her accomplishments by awarding her an honorary Doctor of Science degree, the first School of Pharmacy graduate to be so honored.

"Responsibility" would be an appropriate middle name for Felice Joseph, whose professional career has been replete with positions of authority in the 23 years since receiving a Bachelor of Science degree from the WVU School of Pharmacy in 1985. Born into a family of pharmacists, Felice can't remember when she first decided to join the profession, simply saying, "It was many, many years ago." The first seven years after graduation she was employed in the outpatient pharmacies at Ruby Memorial Hospital in Morgantown and at the Charleston Area Medical Center (Memorial Division and Women's and Children's Hospital) in Charleston. However, as time passed and drug prices escalated, Felice began to notice disquiet and public displeasure that had been absent in the earlier years of her practice. She decided to leave hospital outpatient pharmacy for a retail position as manager of a chain store pharmacy. Looking back to the early years of her varied pharmacy experiences, Felice most enjoyed compounding pharmacy practice, the manufacture of intravenous solutions for a home healthcare agency, and providing supplies to various outpatient surgery centers.

In 1998, Felice accepted a position with the State as a director in the West Virginia Public Employees Insurance Agency (PEIA), where her primary responsibility has been oversight of the prescription drug program for a population of almost 200,000 people. Her position brings her in contact not only with the insured and providers, but also with those who require interaction with the PEIA Finance Board, legislators, and their staffs. Today, she is the lead person at PEIA for the Retiree Drug Subsidy (RDS) program with Medicare Part D and for 35,000 Medicare primary PEIA retirees. Felice's duties include working with The Pharmacy Workgroup and

RXIS, a multi-state purchasing group. Her performance with this group has been recognized as outstanding, resulting in receipt of the 2003 and 2004 Innovations Awards. These awards recognize innovation in State government by West Virginia Multi-State Pharmacy Benefit Management Services of the Council of State Governments. Felice's publications have appeared in journals pertinent to her profession.[18]

Analogous to Felice Joseph's unique position in state government, Elizabeth Kniska Keyes has an equally prominent position at the national level. After Elizabeth graduated with a Bachelor of Science in pharmacy degree from West Virginia University in 1991, she acquired a baccalaureate degree in biology with a minor in technical writing from Wheeling Jesuit University. She then completed the Executive Management Program for Pharmacy Leaders at the Wharton School of Business at the University of Pennsylvania. During her subsequent 13 years as an executive at APhA, Elizabeth has been instrumental in creating a large number of tools and resources for pharmacist-centered vaccine administration and immunization promotion. Elizabeth is a leader in developing premier immunization certificate training programs for pharmacists, with the "Pharmacy-Based-Immunization Delivery" program officially recognized by the Centers for Disease Control and Prevention since 1998. This program is now the standard training curriculum for pharmacists and student pharmacists nationwide.

Elizabeth's current title is Vice President of Strategic Alliances and Business Development at the APhA in Washington, D.C. In this position she is responsible for the operation of key APhA business units, namely business and grant development, meetings and expositions, education and training, and strategic alliances and federal programs. Elizabeth oversees partnerships and alliances with healthcare stakeholder groups to advance the Association's patient care initiatives and business agenda. In addition, Elizabeth creates strategies to market APhA's education and communication capabilities to key pharmaceutical manufacturers and develops projects and opportunities to promote the professional services of pharmacists. She is also responsible for the development and implementation of home study monographs, scientific symposia, and educational conferences for APhA. On the local level, Elizabeth has served as president of the WVU School of Pharmacy Alumni Association and is a member of the School of Pharmacy Board of Advisors.

An exponent of effective pharmacy administration, Peggy A. King is currently Pharmacy Unit Director at the Department of Health and Human

Resources, Bureau for Medical Services of the West Virginia Medicaid program. Over her nine years of service to West Virginia, Peggy has directed the development and implementation of policies that relate to pharmacy benefits for the 350,000 members of the state Medicaid program.

A native of Chesapeake, Ohio, Peggy obtained her pre-pharmacy education at Marshall University and a Bachelor of Science in pharmacy degree from The Ohio State University in 1972. Among her many accomplishments are the implementation of a Preferred Drug List, a State Maximum Allowable Cost program for generic drugs, and the implementation of a new pharmacy point-of-sale processing system that has been certified by the federal government's Centers for Medicare and Medicaid Services. Peggy is the Bureau's liaison with the West Virginia Board of Pharmacy and professional associations and carries out the monumental task of educating state legislators on pharmacy related issues.

A major contributor to effective pharmacy practice at West Virginia University hospitals is clinician, educator, and administrator Carol Woodward. She has implemented pediatric pharmacy, adult critical care, and operating room services in her tenure as Director of Pharmacy Services at Ruby Memorial Hospital. Utilizing her management skills, Carol has assisted in the implementation of computerized physician order entry and automated dispensing systems using unit-based cabinets and robotics.

Carol currently serves in the American Society of Health-System Pharmacists House of Delegates. She has served the WVU School of Pharmacy as a Clinical Assistant Professor and as a member of the School's executive committee. Carol received her Bachelor of Science in pharmacy from West Virginia University and Doctor of Pharmacy degree from the University of North Carolina and has completed an ASHP-Accredited Residency in Clinical Hospital Pharmacy at West Virginia University Hospitals. She is a fellow of the Wharton Executive Management Program of the University of Pennsylvania.

Carol's management skills have not gone unrecognized. She is a recipient of the WVU School of Medicine's Award for Excellence in Clinical Practice. She recently received the ASHP Executive Vice President's Award for Courageous Service for her work associated with Hurricane Katrina disaster relief at Camp Dawson in Preston County.

Many present day pharmacists recall the cigarette commercial a few years back with the tag line, "You've come a long way, baby!" Considering Willa Hood Strickler and her dogged determination to practice her profession, that commercial was indeed a remarkable understatement for pharmacy. Willa was ahead of her time since nearly two decades elapsed before Alice Bennett stepped forward as the second of her gender to take a prominent place in the profession. Dean Lester Hayman also deserves credit for having the foresight to realize that pharmacy was an ideal profession for women, although he was known to say, "Women make the best pharmacists because they are the better housekeepers."[19] It is unfortunate that so few are alive who recall his determination to have three women per class at a time when female enrollment ranged from zero to two (Table 1). It is doubtful that even he dreamed of a day when the majority of pharmacy graduates would be women, a trend that continues today and presumably into the future.

Table 1

Gender of West Virginia
Pharmacy Graduates in the 1940s

Year	No. of Graduates	Male	Female
1940	7	5	2
1941	8	8	0
1942	14	14	0
1943	11	11	0
1944	4	4	0
1945	4	2	2
1946	5	2	3
1947	10	8	2
1948	26	19	7
1949	32	27	5

Part Five

Moving on and Beyond

Chapter Thirteen

Changing Roles and Responsibilities

In an informal survey of West Virginia pharmacists who have changed careers and their stated reasons for change, few surprises were encountered. Most of those interviewed had built on their pharmacy education to enter patient-care related fields such as medicine or dentistry, while a lesser number diverged to the basic sciences where they became recognized for research on novel therapies for diseases such as AIDS or cancer. Pharmacy is a discipline in which knowledge gained can be utilized to further develop a career choice. Even pharmacists who chose law as a career tended to select a branch of law where their pharmacy background would be of value. Common to these individuals was their use of pharmacy as a cornerstone on which to build a career, rather than as a steppingstone to change.

In a 41-year span of time from 1965 through 2006, 96 of the 2,720 WVU pharmacy graduates (3.5%) are known to have made career changes that materially affected their lives, with the largest number becoming physicians (Table 1). Although the data are incomplete, this is still a very small percentage of the pharmacy graduates. Of interest, most of these pharmacists first considered a career change after building a successful pharmacy practice. Michael Cunningham is an example of those pharmacists who changed careers to become physicians.

Michael Edward Cunningham is a pharmacist-physician who was born in Paden City, West Virginia, on August 31, 1952. After enrolling in the West Virginia University general studies program in 1970, his roommate, a pre-pharmacy major, convinced Mike that pharmacy was the profession for him. Mike had never given pharmacy or medicine a thought prior to that time. After considering his roommate's suggestion, Mike switched his major to the pre-pharmacy program and was accepted by the School of Pharmacy two years later. He thrived academically and was elected to membership in the Rho Chi Honor Society in his third year. Mike graduated *Magna Cum Laude* in 1975.

On completing his internship, Mike practiced hospital pharmacy at Ohio Valley Hospital in Wheeling, West Virginia, for three years. It was there that he developed an interest in medicine and was urged by several friends to apply to medical school. As Mike gained experience in the general field of medicine and learned what was required of a physician, he began to seriously consider the career change. The stress of long hours of study to acquire a medical education concerned Mike, but he felt he was up to the challenge. Besides, there was not much room for advancement in hospital pharmacy in those days. Reflecting back to his decision to enter medicine, Mike emphasizes he was not dissatisfied with pharmacy, but rather medicine offered a challenge he wanted to meet. Should he fail, he would be content to return to pharmacy practice. Rather than apply to several medical schools as some of his acquaintances did, Mike applied to only one and if not accepted, he rationalized, he would return to the practice of pharmacy. However, his future fate awaited him as Mike was accepted to the West Virginia University School of Medicine in 1978. Mike excelled in medical school as he had studying pharmacy. Upon graduation, he was accepted into an obstetrics and gynecology residency program at Akron City Hospital in Ohio, although family considerations prompted a change to radiology within a year. However, Mike soon realized he had a conflict; radiology as a specialty was not very fulfilling to someone with his gregarious personality. Thus, Mike selected ultrasonography as a subspecialty because it involved obstetrics that he truly enjoyed, and it provided greater patient contact than radiology.

Mike has been Ultrasound Section Chief at West Virginia University Hospitals since 1998 and is highly regarded as a teacher by the obstetric residents. Mike is extensively involved in the University's radiology outreach program, holds an appointment as clinical associate professor of radiology at the West Virginia School of Osteopathic Medicine, and is also a consultant at St. Joseph Hospital in Buckhannon.[1] Mike has achieved the degree of satisfaction he anticipated from medicine but admits it has created more moments of stress than he would have experienced as a pharmacist. Interestingly, Mike credits his experience in pharmacy with enabling him to endure that stress. Mike practiced pharmacy through medical school, but voluntarily surrendered his pharmacy license in 2000 when he felt too removed from pharmacy to safely practice.

Judie Charlton is another physician who was first a pharmacist. Reared in Fairmont, West Virginia, her grandmother and family physician both encouraged her to attend pharmacy school, having witnessed the proliferation of new drug entities entering the marketplace following World War II. During her senior year of high school, the Fairmont General Hospital staff went on strike, causing a major disruption of medical care for Marion County. Judie volunteered her services to the hospital in whatever capacity she could be used. She was started in the laundry and then transferred to central supply. Her ability to remember medication names was noted by the staff, so Judie was moved to the hospital pharmacy. Throughout pharmacy school, Judie returned each summer to Fairmont General's inpatient pharmacy. Not only did she enjoy working in the pharmacy, but the money earned helped defray college expenses.

However, in her senior year of pharmacy school Judie realized what she enjoyed most was being part of the hospital medical team. She particularly enjoyed helping the team select the drugs to be used (for in-patient care) rather than compounding or dispensing. Judie applied for admission to medical school and in 1980 enrolled in the WVU School of Medicine. Judie believes her pharmacy education prepared her for medical school by not only providing knowledge of medications, but also how to work in the hospital system from a business perspective. Like Michael Cunningham, much of Judie's professional time is spent teaching medical students and residents. Judie considers her pharmacy background not only a huge asset when she entered medicine but it continues to be of value today in her career as an ophthalmologist who specializes in the treatment of glaucoma.[2] She is currently professor and chair of the Department of Ophthalmology at WVU.

A third pharmacist-physician selected a path less frequently traveled to make a unique career change. After receiving his Bachelor of Science degree in pharmacy from WVU in 1953, Jimmie L. Mangus obtained a medical doctor degree from the Medical College of Virginia in 1959 and entered government service in 1967 as medical director of the fledgling Medicaid program with the West Virginia Department of Welfare, Division of Medical Care Standards. Jimmie ran the Medicaid program until he retired from government service in March 1994. At the Department of Welfare, Mangus organized the program that became one of the nation's premier health programs. After retiring from the Department of Welfare, Jimmie became vice president for medical affairs for the Charleston Area Medical Center, a position he held until he again retired in 1999.[3]

Robert James Beto II is another pharmacist-physician who has made several career changes that augment one another. A son of a high school football coach, Bob's initial focus was on sports. He attended West Virginia

Wesleyan College on football and baseball scholarships, but his interests gradually changed as he became more and more involved with chemistry and biology. Following receipt of a Bachelor of Science degree in biology in 1983, he studied biochemistry at West Virginia University for a year and applied for admission to pharmacy school. Bob planned to follow in the footsteps of a pharmacist relative, much to the consternation of his father who wanted him to become a state policeman. Once in pharmacy school, Bob couldn't get enough pharmacology and physiology to satisfy his interest in the biomedical sciences. His desire to learn diagnostics and pharmacotherapy were such that thoughts of medical school entered his mind. Bob practiced pharmacy for a year to help him decide whether to remain in pharmacy or become a physician. He selected medicine. Bob applied to the Marshall University and West Virginia University medical schools, was accepted by both, and in 1993 he received an M.D. degree from WVU. A residency in internal medicine followed, as did a fellowship in cardiology. Today, Bob serves as chief of the Cardiology Section of the Department of Medicine at WVU, with an academic rank of assistant professor. He is nationally recognized as an authority on interventional cardiology.[4]

Law is second only to medicine as the choice of pharmacists who make a career change. Notable examples of West Virginia pharmacists who later became attorneys include Brian Gallagher, Stephen Brooks, Karen Kahle, and Andrea Miller. Brian Gallagher obtained a Bachelor of Science degree in pharmacy from West Virginia University School of Pharmacy in 1981, followed by a law degree from Wake Forest University in 1984. Rather than distance himself from pharmacy practice, Brian combined the two professions through a focus on litigation, health, and corporate law. He has had an active and rewarding professional career. Currently serving as vice president of regulatory compliance for the Rite Aid Corporation, Brian was previously vice president for risk management and governance for NDCHealth and General Counsel for TechRx, Incorporated, the nation's leading pharmacy software company. He has also been director of pharmacy regulatory affairs for the National Association of Chain Drug Stores (NACDS), where he interfaced with Congress, federal regulatory agencies, state legislatures and boards of pharmacy. Prior to his association with NACDS, Brian was general counsel for West Virginia University Hospitals where he was responsible for legal affairs. He also served eight years in the West Virginia House of Delegates where he addressed a wide range of concerns, including being involved in a revision of the Pharmacy Practice Act. Brian remains an adjunct faculty member of the Department of Pharmaceutical Systems and Policy of the West Virginia University School of Pharmacy.[5]

Stephen Brooks is a pharmacist-attorney who is no longer active in the practice of pharmacy. Stephen graduated from the WVU School of Pharmacy in 1971, following which he received a Doctor of Jurisprudence degree from the WVU College of Law in 1975. Brooks is a trial lawyer who practices in professional liability (malpractice) cases, defending hospitals, physicians, and other hospital professionals. As an undergraduate pharmacy student, his mentor, Dean Raphael Bachmann, encouraged him to study law after graduating from pharmacy school with a goal of working in the pharmaceutical industry. Instead, for a year after graduating, Steve served as a staff pharmacist for a pharmacy chain. However, he found the routine nature of his day-to-day practice non-challenging and decided he needed a career change. Having a military obligation to fulfill, active duty in the army provided Steve with time to contemplate his future plans. After separation from the service, Steve enrolled in law school. It was in law school at West Virginia University that Steve realized his communication skills were best adapted to the courtroom. Thus, he has been a trial lawyer since graduating. According to Steve, the training he received in pharmacy school prepared him to communicate with other professionals, particularly those in scientific and health care fields, which helped him understand complex issues and translate them into language a jury can understand.[6]

Karen E. Kahle graduated from the West Virginia University School of Pharmacy in 1982 and practiced pharmacy from 1982 to 1987. Karen then studied law at the West Virginia University College of Law from 1987 to 1990 and began her legal career in 1990. Like Brian Gallagher, Karen taught pharmacy law at the School of Pharmacy for her first five years as an attorney, but has not practiced pharmacy since graduating from law school. Karen's practice is devoted to litigation as a defense attorney, often representing hospitals, physicians, dentists, and other health care practitioners. Reflecting back on her career, Karen was frustrated that she was only infrequently called upon to utilize her medical knowledge as a pharmacist. As a defense attorney, she frequently uses her medical background to prepare a defense in a medical liability case.[7] Law and pharmacy actually have a common denominator: both disciplines require extensive use of communication skills.

Andrea Miller is a pharmacist-attorney who has made a successful career in regulatory affairs. Born in 1966, Andrea graduated from the WVU

School of Pharmacy in 1989. Andrea enrolled in pharmacy school because of her interest in health care, and chemistry was her first love in high school. She recalls sitting through a lecture by WVU faculty member Dr. Paula Jo Stout about the National Pharmaceutical Council Internship Program and thought to herself, "What kind of a 'Geek' would want to do that?" only to find herself as 'that Geek' the next year. By graduation, Andrea had decided product development (formulations) in industry was the career of choice for her. Andrea was impressed by the team effort employed at Mylan Pharmaceuticals that differed so much from the solitary approach to the practice of pharmacy; she considered this an opportunity to grow and learn from other professionals. In her mind, formulations represented the true compounding of modern pharmacy. After passing her licensing exam in 1989, she accepted employment at Mylan where she has remained ever since. However, Andrea developed an interest in regulatory affairs, and in 1993 applied to the WVU College of Law. Working part time, she finished first in her law school class in 1999. Today, Andrea serves as vice president of regulatory affairs at Mylan Pharmaceuticals.[8]

As previously noted, an ability to communicate is vitally important to the practicing pharmacist. With the exception of this need to communicate, pharmacy and the ministry have little in common. Despite a paucity of similarities, five of West Virginia's well-known and highly successful ministers have had a career in both disciplines. The Reverend Lloyd Courtney, pastor of Lewisburg's Old Stone Presbyterian Church, was a pharmacist prior to entering the ministry.[9] However, after becoming ordained, Lloyd no longer practiced pharmacy. The Reverend John Cooper-Martin of Point Pleasant, West Virginia, a 1976 alumnus of the WVU School of Pharmacy, practiced pharmacy for nine years before entering the ministry. Enrolling in the seminary in 1985, John obtained a master's degree in pastoral counseling from Catholic University in Washington, D.C. and was ordained in the United Church of Christ three years later. He now lives in Rockville, Maryland, with a ministry of pastoral counseling.[10]

In contrast to Courtney and Cooper-Martin who left pharmacy after becoming ordained, three other pharmacists have developed a harmonious dual practice of the disciplines. Donald Sinclair of Bethlehem, West Virginia, received a Bachelor of Science degree in pharmacy in 1957, following which he earned a Master of Arts degree in bible philosophy from the American Bible Institute. He served as a lay minister of the Methodist Church throughout his years of pharmacy practice and also served as mayor (see Chapter 3). Isadore R. Wein, a prominent Beckley rabbi, surpassed Courtney and Sinclair by practicing both community and hospital pharmacy while providing rabbinical services for southern West Virginia (see Chapter 11). Likewise, Michael J. Krupa graduated from the WVU School of Pharmacy in 1973 and practiced pharmacy in Buckhannon and Morgantown before opening his own pharmacy, the Professional Rx Shoppe, in Harrisville, West Virginia. Despite a successful practice with ownership of his own pharmacy, after 11 years as a pharmacist Mike made a life-changing decision to enter the ministry. He entered Asbury Theological Seminary in Wilmore, Kentucky, and graduated with a Master of Divinity degree three years later. Mike appreciated Asbury's evangelical thrust and remained with the institution after graduation to serve as its director of development. He has traveled extensively as a missionary to places as far away as Argentina as part of an 18-member health care-ministry team, where Mike practiced both disciplines in rural, underserved areas. Mike characterizes pharmacy and the ministry as "a nice blend," having maintained his pharmacy license through the years. Today, he is a teaching and counseling pastor who has his own church and continues to practice pharmacy. With pride, Mike says he has been involved with pharmacy since the fifth grade and knew by the eighth grade he wanted to be a pharmacist. Mike has derived equal satisfaction through his work in both professions.[11]

In contrast to the differences between pharmacy and the ministry, research and pharmacy form a natural duet. Doctors Frank Lilly, Anna Calcagno, Paula Jo Stout, and Alice Pau are extraordinary examples of pharmacists who became research scientists. They differ in that Drs. Calcagno, Stout, and Pau maintain an active pharmacy license; Dr. Lilly never renewed his pharmacy license once it expired. Each has achieved national recognition by utilizing their pharmacy education to enhance their research careers.

Frank Eugene Lilly was a nationally renowned scientist known for his AIDS related work although, regrettably, his sexual orientation predominated over his scientific achievements. Born in

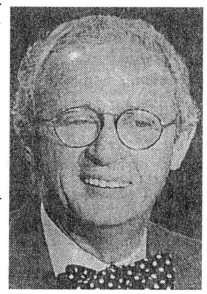

Frank Lilly

Charleston, West Virginia, in 1930, Frank received a Bachelor of Science degree in pharmacy from the West Virginia University School of Pharmacy in 1951.[12] As an undergraduate, he was elected to membership in Phi Lambda Upsilon Honorary Chemical Society, a harbinger of his future life as a scientist.[13] Following two years of service in the U.S. Army, Frank returned to Charleston in 1953 to practice pharmacy but soon decided the profession was not for him.[14] When his license lapsed in 1954, Frank decided to pursue a Ph.D. degree in organic chemistry from the University of Paris, which he received in 1959.[12] By the time Frank joined the genetics department at Albert Einstein College of Medicine as a research fellow in 1965, he had seven publications in prestigious journals such as *Science* and *The Lancet*.

Frank's first research was conducted at the Memorial Sloan-Kettering Cancer Center where he discovered a previously unknown virus. Due to his tremendous potential, his collaborators encouraged Frank to pursue a Ph.D. in biology and genetics, a quest that culminated in 30 years of investigation of retroviruses and genetic patterns of resistance to cancer in mice. In 1983, Frank was elected to membership in the National Academy of Sciences. Six years later he was named Professor of Molecular Genetics and chairman of that department at Einstein College, where he served until retirement.[12]

Frank's first personal encounter with AIDS occurred when a graduate student in the genetics department at Einstein College died of the disease. In 1984, Frank was appointed to serve on the board of the Gay Men's Health Crisis group, a private AIDS support and advocacy organization that provided services to individuals with AIDS in New York. However, he left that board in 1986, having little interest in advocacy organizations. The following year Frank was appointed by President Ronald Reagan to the newly formed Presidential Commission on Human Immunodeficiency Virus (HIV) Epidemic.[12]

The Commission was created by an executive order of President Reagan on June 24, 1987, with a scientific rather than a political agenda. Mrs. Reagan, the President's most influential and trusted advisor, handpicked Frank for precisely what he was, an expert on retroviruses and not an AIDS advocate.[15] However, Frank represented a compromise candidate who might be satisfactory to both scientists and activists.[16] On accepting the appointment to the panel, Dr. Lilly pledged "to forcefully represent the gay community as well as the biomedical community," a statement intended to mollify the AIDS activists who wanted a politically, rather than scientifically, oriented panel. These activists were not easily mollified, though. When Frank left the Gay

Men's Health Crisis group, a co-founder of the group stated that Dr. Lilly was "more in sympathy with his friends at the National Institutes of Health rather than with the gay community." [17]

President Reagan's 12-member Commission intended to eliminate the deadly disease, analogous to smallpox and polio. The Commission included John Cardinal O'Connor, leader of the Archdiocese of New York; Dr. Lilly; Penny Pullen, an Illinois legislator who advocated mandatory premarital testing; and, in the words of *New York Times* columnist Philip Boffey, "other members who are not prominent in the AIDS field," a polite way of saying these individuals had little if any experience with AIDS.[18] The composition of the Commission was not well received by either the medical community or the press. Although prominent and well credentialed in various medical fields, none of the members with the exception of Dr. Lilly were AIDS experts. The press also considered Dr. Lilly the most controversial appointee: conservatives wanted no gay or AIDS infected individuals on the Commission while AIDS advocates wanted to be well represented. A prominent Republican senator, quoted in the *New York Times,* said the White House should not have appointed Dr. Lilly to the Commission "to avoid sending the message to society, especially to impressionable youth, that homosexuality is simply an alternative lifestyle." [18] In contrast, the dean of the Albert Einstein College of Medicine lauded Frank's appointment to the panel. Dean Dominick P. Purpura considered Frank well qualified and ideal for the Commission. Dr. Purpura described Frank as a scientist who combined the talent of a classical geneticist with an innovative mastery of the most sophisticated concepts and methodologies of immunology and molecular biology. [19]

The Presidential Commission held its organizational meeting in September 1987. The members heard from more than a dozen individuals representing minority groups and intravenous drug abusers, as well as those distressed with the Commission's composition. In particular, the Commission's composition was criticized for the absence of "those infected with AIDS." To help address the concerns of the assembly, Dr. Lilly questioned the absence on the program of interest groups representing homosexuals, which was met with enthusiastic applause.[20] Frank also addressed the problem of "AIDS-related discrimination" because it was not generally known to exist, and he emphasized the need for more public leadership and increased efforts to develop effective drug therapies." [21]

Barely a month passed before a second crisis confronted the panel. The chairman and vice chairman of the Commission resigned, citing infighting and ideological differences among the panel members that made their work impossible.[22] The new chairman selected was a retired admiral and former Chief of Naval Operations.[22] By adapting his leadership skills to the AIDS epidemic, the admiral, who lacked both medical education and experience with the disease, quickly became a proponent of aggressive AIDS diagnosis and management. Under this new leadership, the Commission made several endorsements and recommendations, including reporting for tracking purposes all who test positive for HIV infection, requiring public health officials to notify sexual partners of infected people who are unwilling to do so themselves, and considering new laws that would criminalize intentional transmission of the AIDS virus. Gradually, the public's perception of the AIDS panel changed. According to the *New York Times,* "President Reagan's AIDS Commission, once derided by critics as incompetent, poorly managed and biased toward a right-wing agenda, has suddenly emerged as a bold, decisive champion of government spending to help the victims of the disease." [23]

Frank had at one point contemplated resigning from the AIDS panel. As he viewed the problem, it would become his responsibility to educate his colleagues about the disease. Likewise, his fellow commissioners did not fully appreciate the civil-rights concerns of the AIDS victims. There was also the matter of public education; the majority of the American public did not understand AIDS. There was a proliferation of AIDS advocacy groups, which were often very vocal and demanding. Frank further felt the President had shown little interest in hearing the gay community's concerns about the disease. Overall, service on the Commission appeared to Frank to be a thankless task. On the other hand, Frank realized he was likely the only panel member who really understood AIDS as a disease process. Thus, his sense of responsibility compelled him to continue. In 1987, Frank was appointed co-president of the Commission, an excellent choice since the admiral's leadership and organizational skills were complemented by Frank's scientific knowledge. Frank retained his position on the Commission and became active in AIDS education.[24]

A third crisis for the President's Commission arose in March 1992. That month the quintessential medical journal, *Rolling Stone Magazine,* published an article suggesting that a Philadelphia medical researcher may have accidentally initiated the AIDS epidemic in the Belgium Congo, now Zaire, in the 1950s. According to *Rolling Stone,* the virus may have been transmitted to the population of Zaire in 1957 during trials of an oral polio vaccine, a vaccine made from monkey kidneys. Frank was part of the six-member committee investigating the report's credibility and disputed the assertion. By announcing there was "almost incontrovertible" evidence that AIDS existed in Africa before the oral polio trials began, he nullified public apprehension regarding oral polio vaccine in the western world. Frank reported that the earliest documented case of AIDS was a merchant seaman who was symptomatic with AIDS in 1958 and died in England in 1959. That seaman had traveled to Africa in 1955 but returned to England in 1957, prior to the beginning of the oral polio trials.[25]

Frank Lilly died of prostate cancer October 14, 1995.[26] Beyond his role as a scientist, Frank's service on the Commission helped address the civil rights concerns of AIDS victims, including inappropriate discrimination. His work touched thousands and made a momentous difference in the lives of many Americans.

In 1993, at the same time that Dr. Lilly was battling his illness, a young future researcher named Anna Maria Calcagno received a Bachelor of Science in pharmacy degree from West Virginia University. Deciding early in the educational process that she wished to pursue a research career, her mentor, WVU faculty member Dr. Paula Stout, helped Anna obtain one of the first internships at Mylan Laboratories in Morgantown. She worked there with several individuals who guided and encouraged her towards her research goal. Anna then attended the University of Michigan where she received a master's degree in pharmaceutics.

Family problems at this time led to a three-year hiatus in Anna's education. Taking time off from her studies, she worked at Wheeling Hospital and a retail pharmacy chain before enrolling in the pharmaceutical chemistry program at the University of Kansas. Anna's interest in the biology of pharmacy rather than its chemistry influenced her to consider the Kansas Ph.D. program, particularly because they had both a pharmaceutical chemistry and a biotechnology program. At Kansas, Anna obtained a National Institutes of Health training grant with an industrial internship at Pharmacia and received her doctorate in 2003. Anna then accepted a post-doctoral fellowship at St. Jude Children's Hospital for a year, when a position at the National Cancer Institute (NCI) became available. At NCI she holds a three-year Pharmacology Research Associate Training (PRAT) fellowship and worked with the cutting edge research leaders in the field of multi-drug resistance. The PRAT fellowship is available only to NIH postdoctoral fellows with a pharmacology background who plan to continue a career in research at the National Cancer Institute. Anna's pharmacy background provided excellent preparation for her research in drug resistance, cancer, and the various disease processes that she now encounters at NIH.[27]

Having mentored Anna Marie Calcagno as a student, it is not surprising that Paula Jo Stout's career parallels Anna Marie's in many respects. Paula Jo graduated from West Virginia University School of Pharmacy in 1978, where she was in the first pharmacy Ph.D. class. After receiving a doctorate in 1986, she joined the Department of Basic Pharmaceutical Sciences at the School as its only female faculty member at that time (she is currently one of only two women in that department). Paula pursued a career in the area of drug delivery by developing safe and effective dosage forms, and by optimizing those formulations and assessing dosage forms, in particular for nutraceuticals, vitamins and herbal products. Early in Paula's career she investigated the quality of drug performance and drug performance failures, especially of herbal products. More recently she has focused on drug delivery of sustained release products in collaboration with the Chemical Engineering Department at WVU, the targeted delivery of antibiotics in collaboration with the WVU School of Dentistry, and the area of sterile injectable products with the pharmaceutical industry (Eli Lilly). She currently works with ophthalmic manufacturers on targeting drugs in ophthalmic preparations.[28]

Paula Jo Stout has an additional area of expertise that is unequaled in West Virginia and undoubtedly many other parts of the country. Antedating to her high school days, she was a twirler at sporting events, and she was a feature twirler while a student at WVU. She continues to use this expertise at West Virginia University to help train the next generation of twirlers to perform at Mountaineer football games.

Another former West Virginian to choose a career in research is Alice Pau. Alice is a staff scientist in the Division of Clinical Research at the NIH's National Institute of Allergy and Infectious Diseases (NIAID). After receiving an undergraduate pharmacy degree from the University of Houston and a Doctor of Pharmacy degree from the University of Michigan, Alice taught at the West Virginia University School of Pharmacy for several years, followed by work as a faculty member at the University of Illinois at Chicago College of Pharmacy. Alice ultimately left Chicago to accept a position as a staff scientist at NIH. At NIAID, she develops guidelines for the use of antiretroviral agents in HIV infected adolescents and adults and prepares guidelines for treating HIV associated opportunistic infections.[29] Alice travels extensively around the globe, particularly to South Africa, to assist in the fight against AIDS.

In contrast to its scientific orientation, pharmacy practice also requires skills in sales, marketing, and entrepreneurship. Valerie Schmidt Mondelli is an individual who successfully employs these skills. Valerie graduated with a Bachelor of Science degree in pharmacy from WVU in 1996. Subsequently armed with an MBA degree, she is now a sales and marketing executive with Per-Se Technologies (formerly NDCHealth) where she is a vice president for pharmacy services and sales in Atlanta. Valerie joined Per-Se/NDCHealth in January 2004. Per-Se provides technology applications and software systems to physician offices, hospitals, health plans and pharmacies. Most pharmacies consider Per-Se/NDCHealth to be a "switch" or network that routes the claim from the pharmacy to the third party payer or health plan. However, Per-Se/NDCHealth also edits claims before they are routed through the network by: 1) prompting the pharmacist to add additional information or correct errors, 2) maximizing reimbursement to the pharmacy and 3) ensuring the claim is in compliance with third party or government requirements. In addition, Per-Se sells practice management software systems, excluding computers, used by pharmacists to fill prescriptions. As vice president, Valerie manages a team of executives who sell new technology products and services to health plans and pharmacy benefits management clients such as Walgreens and Kroger. She personally manages their two largest accounts, CVS and Wal-Mart, and travels extensively throughout the nation to meet with customers. Working closely with the product management and operations groups, Valerie uses feedback regarding the needs of her clientele to create new solutions for their problems.[30]

Jann Burks Skelton, like Valerie Mondelli, is another sales and marketing executive headquartered in metropolitan Atlanta. Jann, a 1991 graduate of the WVU School of Pharmacy, operates Silver Pennies Consulting, LLC, a healthcare consulting company that works with the pharmaceutical industry, managed care groups, and healthcare organizations to develop and implement direct-to-the-patient market strategies. She designs and markets customized solutions for the entire health care supply chain from the manufacturer to the wholesaler, hospital, or practitioner.[31]

Thomas E. Menighan graduated with a Bachelor of Science in pharmacy degree from WVU in 1974 and earned an MBA from Averett College in Richmond, VA, in 1990 (see Chapter 10). Tom is an entrepreneur who founded eight corporations or partnerships, of which he has sold three. Currently, Tom is general manager of Integrity Solutions Division of Health Pathways in the Washington, D.C., area, a company that satisfies a growing need for pharmaceutical supply chain integrity by the efficient provision of pharmaceuticals and consumer health care information. His company provides services and systems to pharmaceutical manufacturers, distributors, and pharmacies in the eastern Unites States. Tom founded and is president of Syn Tegra, LLC, in Germantown, Maryland, a company that serves clients in the areas of risk management, 340B Systems, anti-counterfeiting, supply chain integrity, and technology of medication information. Additionally, he developed CornerDrugStore.com.,© managed the PharMark Corporation — the creator of RationalMed©— and licensed systems for states to conduct drug utilization reviews for Medicaid enrollees.[32] These achievements to date along with those described previously, exceed what most pharmacists accomplish in their entire career.[33]

Michele Vigneault McNeill is an exceptional role model as an entrepreneur and an outstanding citizen. She founded and operated a financially successful business with an unfaltering focus on her clients, frequently patients with life-threatening diseases. McNeill received a bachelor's degree in pharmacy from West Virginia University in 1975, where she was elected president of the Rho Chi Honor Society. After earning a Doctor of Pharmacy degree, she completed a residency in hospital pharmacy practice at Mercy Hospital in Pittsburgh, PA.

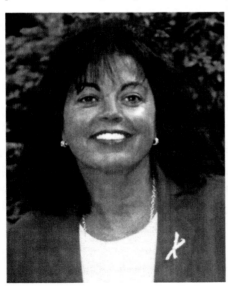

Michele V. McNeill

In 1988, Michele founded Kern McNeill International (KMI), a contract research organization providing clinical drug development services to research-based pharmaceutical manufacturers (see Chapter 12). She was named a Distinguished Alumna of WVU in 1999, received the Distinguished West Virginian Award, and in 2004 was inducted into the West Virginia Business Hall of Fame. Most recently, in 2005 West Virginia University awarded McNeill an honorary Doctor of Science degree.[34]

This chapter has profiled a few of the many individuals who used their pharmacy education and training to pursue related, or in some cases very divergent, professions. Regardless of the path they chose, these professionals were able to accomplish goals in ways they likely never thought possible as pharmacy students. Although not "traditional pharmacists" in the full meaning of the term, each of these individuals is noteworthy in his or her own way and has made a significant contribution to society.

Table 1

Career Changes by West Virginia Pharmacists 1965-2006

Discipline Chosen	Number	Percent*
Medicine	56	2.0
Law	14	0.5
Dentistry	9	0.3
Ministry	5	0.2
Entrepreneur	3	0.1
Scientific Research	4	0.1
Sales and Marketing	2	0.07
Military	1	0.04
Podiatry	1	0.04
Secondary Education	1	0.04
Total	*96*	*3.4*

*Of the number of graduates during this time period

Lessons Learned and Miles To Go...

Marie A. Abate

"...The woods are lovely, dark, and deep,
But I have promises to keep,
And miles to go before I sleep,
And miles to go before I sleep."

Robert Frost, "Stopping by Woods on a Snowy Evening," 1923

History does not simply illustrate where we have been. Rather, it helps explain who we are and serves to guide our future paths. West Virginia pharmacists of the past have played important roles in shaping our current profession. Traits shared by many of these individuals include a pioneer spirit, a refusal to give up in the face of seemingly insurmountable odds, service to others, and heroism. They have left West Virginia pharmacy with a legacy. Although many of their names may be forgotten over time, their accomplishments will endure.

Who would have thought that Robert Fahrrey's opening of the first West Virginia pharmacy in the early 1800s would represent the exploration of unknown territory? Pharmacy practice up to that time involved selling medicines, chemicals, and rather bizarre "home remedies" out of a buckboard or from the back of a horse, which represented delivery service directly to the "patients." In contrast, working from a fixed location where the patients would come to you involved a tremendous risk. This risk proved to be successful, and the number of pharmacies has since exploded. However, history shows that both types of practices can be successful. How can this knowledge help us in the future? As the population ages, greater numbers of patients will reside in assisted living homes or have difficulty traveling to a pharmacy. Future pharmacists will be called upon to function as pioneers once more by exploring new mechanisms for delivering medications directly to where these patients reside. Further, as a result of new federal regulations and in light of growing concerns about medication use safety, the emphasis has gradually shifted from a product-oriented to a service and information-oriented pharmacy profession. As with the other health professions, pharmacists have begun to realize that they cannot advance appropriate medication use in a vacuum. Pharmacy must form closer working partnerships with patients and other health care professionals as part of an integrated team.

The story of William Weiss in Chapter 2 illustrates how the profession has changed over time and how one small town pharmacist, through tremendous ambition, resourcefulness, and a keen business sense, went from selling patent medicines to ownership of a multi-million dollar conglomerate. From the start of his practice as a young man, William had his sights set on higher goals that he ultimately achieved through hard work and collaboration with his friend, Albert Diebold. Although their early technique of marketing one medicine to counteract the negative effects of another is suspect at best, a valuable lesson can be learned from these men: "raise the bar" in practice and never quit working to achieve your goals. However, Weiss' story also tragically shows how bigotry and intolerance can wipe out a lifetime of effort and achievement. Despite a lack of ties or loyalty to Germany, his German ancestry resulted in the United States government seizing his business assets during World War II. It is difficult for those born after the war ended to understand how such an injustice could occur. Surely this will never occur again…or, could it? Prejudice is insidious and pervasive in our current society. As one of the most visible and accessible health professionals for the public, pharmacists must serve as role models of racial and religious tolerance for their patients and communities.

The stories told in the first two chapters of Part Two were inspirational. How did these pharmacists have the time to not only perform their professional duties (several were pharmacy owners) but to also serve on a number of community groups and hold public office at local or state levels? In the small towns where many of the pharmacist-mayors served, their public presence and position of respect as pharmacists blended well with their public servant role. Irrespective of the town size, however, these pharmacists did not take their mayoral responsibilities lightly and worked hard to improve their communities. Although Mayor George Rice was lauded for his efforts following the Shinnston tornado in 1944, his taking upon himself the responsibility of keeping the streets of that town swept and clean for years later is the image best remembered. Why? It illustrates the priorities of all these individuals – professional service, patient service, and community service, with all being equally important. Apparently, these individuals experienced personal satisfaction through giving. Some were also ahead of their time. West Virginia pharmacists just recently obtained the right to administer immunizations. Those who opposed pharmacist-provided immunizations should have looked in the past to Mr. Sinclair. Pharmacist-mayor Donald Sinclair in 1961 prepared and administered polio vaccinations and served a key leadership role in safeguarding his community from that debilitating disease.

Some leaders ultimately become heroes. Such was the case of Ed Rockis, a pharmacist and triple purple heart recipient who, as a company commander under heavy enemy fire during the Korean War, led a rescue mission for several of his stranded men. But Ed was a hero of another sorts as well, to patients who can't speak for themselves – our furry, four-legged companions. Ed established a successful veterinary pharmacy practice that served north central West Virginia. There are also heroes who never thought of themselves as leaders, but their actions and deeds were inspirational to their communities. Charlie Stump was the epitome of this type of hero. He helped people in need by providing them with not only professional support but also with insurance money or donations. Beyond this, though, he gave of his professional time and energy to provide patients with medications after hours whenever needed or when a flood devastated his community. What lessons should be learned from Ed, Charlie, and the other pharmacist heroes described in Chapters 5 and 6? Military personnel and pharmacists share a responsibility to the public, the same as other health professionals. Unfortunately, a number of pharmacy students and pharmacy practitioners over the past several years have placed their needs above those of their patients. How? By not taking the time to fully address patients' concerns, by neglecting to talk to patients about their medications and to reinforce physicians' instructions, by failing to address their own knowledge deficits, or by not accepting responsibility for inactions or inappropriate actions. History has shown a continuing trust by patients in their pharmacists. Pharmacy practitioners need to always remember this trust, and students need to learn the obligations that accompany such trust.

Educating each new class of future pharmacists is a significant responsibility and undertaking. The West Virginia University School of Pharmacy did not have an easy beginning. Beleaguered early faculty member Gordon Bergy not only developed the initial pharmacy curriculum but he taught most of it himself. The first Dean, J. Lester Hayman, had to contend with few faculty teaching large numbers of students in meager facilities. But he understood the importance of service to the extent that he spent summers traveling around the state working in pharmacies. The blend of academician/clinician is especially needed today in pharmacy education. This type of individual has a strong commitment to patient care and clinical teaching. In addition, they nurture in students a questioning mind to continually explore ways to improve patients' health and pharmacy practice. The focus on the student is a theme that runs through the stories of the emeritus faculty described in Chapter 8, with Dr. James Lim perhaps stating it best, "...the respect of a student is the greatest reward a teacher can receive."

Each generation of educators has confronted new problems and unique circumstances that were likely incomprehensible to their predecessors. Who fifty years ago would have envisioned the number of drugs and drug classes that are marketed today? Or, that a significant proportion of the present curriculum would consist of a type of apprenticeship (with its inherent scheduling difficulties) in which students learn by working side by side with pharmacists? Would Professor Geiler in the 1950s have guessed that talking on the phone would become a problem within a classroom or that it would allow students sitting on opposite sides of a classroom to share examination answers? Would he have been surprised to realize that many future patients and health care providers would be unable to describe exactly what a pharmacist does beyond the simple dispensing of drugs?

The former deans and faculty members not only handled the obstacles of their time but made the WVU School of Pharmacy stronger as a result. Research was strengthened, outreach services were initiated, faculty numbers were increased, female students were admitted in increasing proportions along with the hiring of many more women as faculty members, physical facilities were strengthened, and fund raising reached an all time high. Future deans and faculty members will once again need to rise to the occasion to resolve their unique problems through hard work and innovative thinking. They must also take a proactive role in working with professional pharmacy associations and organizations to establish a core set of accepted duties and responsibilities for pharmacists that are consistent across all practice environments and that are clear and accepted by other health care providers and the public. This will be no small undertaking.

Dr. James Beal devoted much personal sacrifice to establish a viable West Virginia professional association in the early 1900s. Why? Dr. Beal understood that a collective strength and vision would more effectively accomplish goals for the profession when compared to individuals working autonomously. The pharmacy profession today is fragmented, particularly at the national level. There are associations for chain drug stores, institutional pharmacies, independent community pharmacies, clinical pharmacy, consultant pharmacy, academic pharmacy, etc. There is no united organization that speaks for all pharmacists and that clearly defines pharmacists' common roles and responsibilities. As a result, many believe that pharmacists simply dispense medications, which in some cases is unfortunately true. Retail pharmacy chains might employ an insufficient number of pharmacists or support staffs for these individuals. This not only prevents these highly educated professionals from fully utilizing their abilities but it promotes errors that can harm patients. Some pharmacists compound the problem because they are only too content to stay behind the counter and fill prescriptions – they fail to keep up with the literature and make little effort to adequately counsel patients. Once again, pharmacy needs to determine how to better work as a unified group to advocate for all members of the profession and guarantee its long-term growth. Is there another as yet unidentified "Dr. Beal" who will step forth to assume this leadership role? Perhaps this individual will come from among those described in the first three chapters of Part Four, the national leaders, regional and local leaders, and current award winners.

The West Virginia pharmacists who became national leaders of pharmacy organizations were high achievers, all of whom implemented or promoted changes to advance the profession. Dr. Cook's devotion to history led to the establishment of the School of Pharmacy's nationally known pharmacy museum. Steve Crawford championed pharmaceutical care provision in small rural hospitals and Tom Menighan advanced home health care and home infusion specialty pharmacy services. John Plummer was an advocate for strong communication skills and patient counseling as well as for better cooperation between state and national pharmacy agencies and organizations. Regionally, the WVPA has been fortunate to have a succession of caring, energetic individuals who led the organization from near bankruptcy to a progressive, cohesive association. In particular, the emergence of strong women to assume the role of president over the past 20 years is a significant departure from the near absolute male dominance in the presidency prior to that time.

Willa Strickler took the bold step in 1907 of being the first woman to apply to and be accepted into the West Virginia Pharmaceutical Association. Alice Bennett was one of the first women to own a pharmacy in West Virginia. Post-World War II, thanks in part to the efforts of Dean Hayman, female student enrollment in pharmacy school increased and never diminished. Chapter 12 describes the careers of several successful women with diverse practice backgrounds who became leaders in their areas. The paths they took that led them to their ultimate destinies were unique and often winding, but they persevered to do what they loved. Pre-dating all of these women was the incomparable Ann Dinardi. Ann Dinardi was a strong woman with a kind heart that she opened to the community within and outside of West Virginia University. As a pharmacy student, she rose above prejudice to her Italian heritage by starting her own sorority open only to Italian women. As a practitioner, Ann became a successful pharmacy businesswoman in the male-dominated profession at that time. She was loved and respected by all who knew her. Although many other women described in Chapter 12 such as Patty Johnston, Elizabeth Scharman, and Michele McNeill have stepped forward to assume important roles in a variety of areas of pharmacy practice and education, women must continue to draw upon their unique skills and talents to serve as leaders and innovators in the profession.

One of the benefits of being a pharmacist is the variety of career options and advancement opportunities available. In addition to the well-known community, hospital, pharmaceutical industry, and academic pharmacist positions, Chapter 13 in Part Five illustrates the stories of several pharmacists who used their training and degree to move on to other areas, within and outside of the profession. Many of these individuals became physicians and found their pharmacy education invaluable in their new careers. The author of this book, Dr. Douglas Glover, is a perfect example of the pharmacist-physician who started his journey as a pharmacist, practiced for most of his life as a devoted obstetrician who also conducted drug-related research, and entered retirement with a focus once again on his beginnings as a pharmacist. Others went on to study law with a focus on medical malpractice, pharmacy law, or pharmacy regulatory affairs. Some emphasized a research or scientist career focused on pharmaceuticals or treatment guideline development.

The commonality in all of the stories told in Part Five, ironically, is their diversity. Medicines and medication use are ubiquitous in our society; thus, many careers and professions can successfully build upon a pharmacy education and training background.

In conclusion, the practice of pharmacy in West Virginia has clearly progressed over the years. However, there is still a long road to travel. This road stretches to the horizon of the next generation and beyond, with bumps to be encountered along the way and unexpected potholes to traverse. Although some predict a gloomy pharmacy future, those dire forecasts have been with us for decades. [1] While no one can accurately predict the future, the miles ahead should ultimately become a pleasing sight in pharmacy's rearview mirror as long as the pharmacists of the future have the strength, courage, and fortitude of their predecessors.

---

1. Stewart RB. *The future of pharmacy: armageddon or pollyanna? Ann Pharmacother* 1995;29:1292-6.

Notes

1. Through the Eyes of Yesterday

1. Roy Bird Cook, *The Annals of Pharmacy in West Virginia* (Charleston, WV: West Virginia State Pharmaceutical Association, 1946)

2. Dennis B. Worthen, *Pharmacy in World War II* (New York: Pharmaceutical Products Press, Haworth Press, Inc., 2004)

3. The University of the Sciences in Philadelphia, ed., *Remington: The Science and Practice of Pharmacy, 21st edition* (Philadelphia: Lippincott Williams & Wilkins, 2005), 14.

2. From a Small Town to the World Stage

1. Marquis Who's Who, *Who's Who in America, 1940-1941* (Chicago: A.N. Marquis, 1941), 21, 2710

2. "Pharmacist Highlights: Boette, Henry O," *The West Virginia Pharmacist* (1953), 6 [1]: 9

3. Charles Mann and Mark Plummer, *The Aspirin Wars* (New York: Alfred A. Knopf, Inc., 1991), 50

4. *Sterling Products, Inc.*, National Park Service, Sec. 8, page 2

5. Mann and Plummer, *The Aspirin Wars*, 51

6. Ibid., 155

7. "Albert Diebold, Drug Leader, Dies," *New York Times*, February 17, 1964

8. Mann and Plummer, *The Aspirin Wars*, 109.

9. Anon. "Dr. Weiss Dies of Crash Injuries," *Wheeling Intelligencer*, September 3, 1942, final edition

10. Mrs. K. Quinn, interview with author, March 8, 2005.

11. Genealogy Division, Stark Country District Library. Canton, Ohio: accessed July 28, 2005.

12. Bill Winsley (Ohio State Board of Pharmacy), interview with author, April 22, 2005.

13. Carol Brown, Jane and Julie Fawcett, interview with author, July 15, 2005.

14. Louis Bockius III, interview with author, July 15, 2005.

15. "Albert Diebold, Drug Leader, Dies," *New York Times*.

16. Mann and Plummer, *The Aspirin Wars*, 5

17. Alfred D. Chandler, Jr., "New Learning at American Home Products," *Harvard Business School Working Knowledge,* April 25, 2005.

18. Anon. "A Foundation for Growth: The Story of the American Home Products Corporation," (American Home Products Corporation, New Jersey), not dated.

19. Anon. "The Sterling Story," (Sterling Drug Company, 1958), 23.

3. *Community Leaders and Mayors*

1. M. Wilson, "His Honor, the Pharmacist," *American Druggist,* 197, 1988, 40-42.

2. Personal Communication, Steve Roberts, Kanawha County Chamber of Commerce, June 16, 2005

3. Obituary of Donald C. Sinclair, *Wheeling Intelligencer,* June 5, 1999.

4. N. Martinez, "The Makings of a Major" (unpublished manuscript), Shepherd University, accessed February 24, 2004.

5. Obituary of Fred C. Allen, *Pocahontas Times,* January 1, 1970.

6. "The Political Graveyard: a Database of Historic Cemeteries," courtesy of Harold M. Forbes, associate curator of the West Virginia and Regional History Collection, Wise Library, West Virginia University.

7. Mrs. L. D. Main, interview with author, June 14, 2005.

8. Richard E. Romig, Jr., interview with author, June 5, 2005.

9. Ibid., June 16, 2005.

10. Mrs. J. L. Turner, interview with author, June 14, 2005.

11. Judy Lawson (Bridgeport City Clerk), interview with author, July 13, 2005.

12. Keith Boggs (Bridgeport City Treasurer), interview with author, August 2, 2005.

13. Paul Turman, Sr., interview with author, July 19, 2005.

14. Dick Jefferson (former council member), interview with author, July 19, 2005.

15. B.J. Payne (Assistant Executive Director of the WV Board of Pharmacy), interview with author, June 2, 2005.

16. J.J. Finlayson, *Shinnston Tornado* (New York: Hobson Book Press, 1946).

17. G.B. Wandell, interview with author, May 31, 2005.

18. Ms. D. Herndon (Shinnston City Clerk), interview with author, May 25, 2005.

19. "Dr. Blissitt Named Mayor of Morgantown," *The West Virginia Pharmacist* (1962), 15 [8]: 9.

20. "Dr. Blissitt to be St. Louis Dean," *The West Virginia Pharmacist* (1964), 17 [3]: 11.

21. Al Carolla, interview with author, August 7, 2006.

4. State Leaders and Legislators

1. *Journal of the American Pharmaceutical Association* (1929), 18 [2], 193

2. *West Virginia Blue Book*, 1955.

3. *History of Pocahontas County* (Marlinton: Pocahontas County Historical Society, 1981), 30.

4. Obituary of Fred C. Allen, *Pocahontas Times*, January 1, 1970.

5. Calvin W. Price, editorial, *Pocahontas Times*, March 12, 1936.

6. Pam Johnson and Vicky Terry, interview with author, June 22, 2006.

7. Courtesy of Harold M. Forbes, associate curator of the West Virginia and Regional History Collection, Wise Library, West Virginia University.

8. Obituary of C. Herbert Traubert, *Wheeling Intelligencer*, December 27, 1987, final edition

9. Paul Glover, "Sheriff's Son is Successor," *Wheeling Intelligencer*, December 27, 1937.

10. Blanche McDowell Neff, "Kindred Kernels," *Wellsburg Daily Herald.* Date unknown, probably printed in February 1938.

11. Dick Traubert, interview with author, April 20, 2006.

12. James Hood, interview with author, April 21, 2006.

13. "One Candidate Follansbee is Proud to Claim," *The Follansbee Review*, date unknown.

14. Obituary of Wendell Traubert, *The Follansbee Review*, undated.

15. "Pat Vale," *Follansbee (WV) Review,* January 6, 1940.

16. John Kirker, "Sen. Traubert Named to 4 Top Committees," *Wheeling Intelligencer*, undated (1949).

17. John Kirker, "Governor Signs Second Bill Filed by Traubert," *Wheeling Intelligencer*, February 26, 1949.

18. D.A. Fleming, J. Grimm, and P. Schumann, *Generation of Growth: A Contemporary View of West Virginia University School of Medicine* (Morgantown, WV: West Virginia University Publication Services, 1990), 4.

19. John M. Slack, "History of the Building Committee in Planning for the West Virginia University Medical Center," typescript, 1976.

20. D.A. Fleming, J. Grimm, and P. Schumann, *Generation of Growth: A Contemporary View of West Virginia University School of Medicine (Morgantown, WV):* West Virginia University Publication Services, 1990), 5.

21. "Herbert Traubert Seeks Re-Election for State Senator – 1st District," undated (1952).

22. John Kirker, "Bill Fought by Traubert," *Wheeling News-Register*, undated.

23. Paul Glover, "New School Aid Plan Presented by Traubert," *Steubenville* (Ohio) *Herald-Star*, undated.

24. John Kirker, "Follansbee Steel Corp to be Moved to Gadsden," *Wheeling Intelligencer*, undated.

25. John Kirker, "Follansbee Steel Hearing Recessed until Monday," *Wheeling Intelligencer*, undated.

26. Telegram from Senator H.M. Kilfore to Herbert Traubert, November 17, 1954.

27. "Santa Comes to Follansbee," *Time Magazine*, December 13, 1954.

28. Dick Traubert, interview with author, May 3, 2006.

29. D.A. Fleming, et. al., *Generation of Growth: A Contemporary View of West Virginia University School of Medicine (Morgantown WV):* West Virginia University Publication Services, School of Medicine, 1990.

30. Dr. Frank O'Connell, interview with author, May 18, 2006.

5. *Behind the Counter to the Front Lines*

1. Wesley F. Craven and James L. Cate, eds., *The Army Air Forces in World War II. Volume II, Europe: Torch to Pointblank* (Chicago: University of Chicago Press, 1949).

2. Curriculum vitae of John J. Halki, M.D., dated August 1, 1999.

3. "A Eulogy for Jack Halki," delivered by Dr. Dennis Barber at a Wright State University Memorial Service, August 4, 2000

4. Obituary of Mary Plummer, *Times West Virginian* (Fairmont), January 26, 2006.

5. Marguerite Higgins, *War in Korea: The Report of a Woman Combat Correspondent* (New York: Garden City, 1951).

6. Knowlton, Leo. Personal communication, March 14, 2006.

7. John Costello, *The Pacific War* (New York: Quill, 1982).

8. "Former WVU Students KIA in World War II." Courtesy of the West Virginia Collection, Wise Library at West Virginia University.

9. After Action Reports for the 358 Infantry Regiment, 90 Inf. Division, RG No. 206, Stack 270, Row 58, Compartment 33, Shelf 2, Box 13395, Located in the National Archives, College Park, Md.

10. Constance Baston of the Charleston (WV) Memorial Monument, interview with author, February 10, 2006.

11. "Lt. Ferguson Killed," *Montgomery News*, July 26, 1944. Provided by Brenda Moore of the Fayette County Library.

12. Gwen Hubbard of the Brooke Country Library in Wellsburg, interview with author, February 12, 2006.

13. Sandy Day, genealogist at the Schiappa Branch of the Public Library of Steubenville and Jefferson County (Ohio), interview with author, February 15, 2006.

14. Obituary of PFC George Rangos, *Steubenville* (Ohio) *Herald-Star*, April 27, 1945.

15. Obituary of Maj. Michael A. Rafferty, *Charleston Gazette*, January 11, 1945.

16. Obituary of Maj. Michael A. Rafferty, *Weston Democrat*, December 22, 1944.

17. "Military Impact of the German V-Weapons," unpublished, courtesy of Dr. Mason R. Schaefer at the U.S. Army Center of Military History, February 9, 2006.

18. Forrest C. Pogue, *George C. Marshall: Education of a General, 1880-1939* (New York: Viking Press, 1967), 227.

19. Merle Miller, *Ike: The Soldier as They Knew Him* (New York: G.P. Putnam's Sons, 1987), 306.

20. Headquarters, West Virginia Military District, Commendation accompanying the Silver Star Medal granted to 1st Lt. Edward W. Rockis, January 11, 1954.

21. Col. Don R. Patton, USAR, personal letter to Mrs. E.W. Rockis, October 31, 2005.

6. Heroes

1. John Finlayson, *Shinnston Tornado*, (New York: Hobson Book Press, 1946).

2. Jim Burks, interview with author, August 8, 2006.

3. Steve Crawford, interview with author, August 28, 2006.

4. Steve Judy, interview with author, August 25, 2006.

5. Milton Proudfoot, interview with author, August 9, 2006.

6. Ruby Baumgartner, interview with author, August 11, 2006

7. Bob Teets and Shelly Long, *Killing Waters* (Terra Alta, W.Va.: Cheat River Publishing, 1985).

8. Eva Burns, interview with author, August 7, 2006.

9. Ethel Lusk, interview with author, August 8, 2006.

10. Al Carolla, interview with author, August 7, 2006.

11. Arvell Wyatt, interview with author, August 7, 2006.

7. Deans

1. Program for the WVU School of Pharmacy Alumni Meeting, June 4, 1961.

2. Rosemary Raczko, Manager of Academic Services, University of Michigan College of Pharmacy, interview with author, September 12, 2005.

3. Anon. "J. Lester Hayman." *The West Virginia Pharmacist* (1963), 16 [7]: 21.

4. Obituary of J. Lester Hayman, *The Dominion Post*, July 7, 1963.

5. Obituary of Raphael O. Bachmann, *The Dominion Post*, December 19, 1972.

6. "Minutemen Organization at WVU," *The West Virginia Pharmacist* (1965), 18 [3]: 12.

7. J.P. Plummer, President's Message, *The West Virginia Pharmacist* (1965), 18 [7]: 3.

8. Office of the Dean, WVU School of Medicine Annual Reports and the Reports of LCME,
   June 1988.

9. "Report of the School of Pharmacy," *The West Virginia Pharmacist* (1966), 9 [1]: 14-17.

10. WVU School of Pharmacy *Showglobe*, (1973), 25 [2]: 1

11. Curriculum vitae of L.A. Luzzi, dated December, 1977.

12. J. Lim, interview with author, June 8, 2005.

13. J.W. Mauger, interview with author, June 7, 2005.

14. J.H. Baldwin, interview with author, August 11, 2005.

15. J.H. Baldwin, interview with author, August 16, 2005.

16. A.I. Jacknowitz, interview with author, June 8, 2005.

17. Curriculum vitae of S.A. Rosenbluth, dated December 30, 1999.

18. Calvin Brister, interview with author, September 22, 2005.

19. J.H. Baldwin, interview with author, August 16, 2005.

20. Curriculum vitae of G.R. Spratto, dated Spring, 2005.

21. G.R. Spratto, interview with author, September 22, 2005.

8. *Emeritus Faculty*

1. Philip B. Covey, ed., *Webster's New International Dictionary*, (Springfield, MA: G&C Merriam Company, 1981).

2. Clarke Ridgway, assistant dean for Student Services, interview with author, December 1, 2006.

3. Robert R. Lewis, interview with author, November 10, 2006.

4. Ann Bond Smith, interview with author, November 10, 2006.

5. Thomas Traubert, interview with author, November 10, 2006.

6. Frank O'Connell, interview with author, November 15, 2006.

7. David Riley, interview with author, December 3, 2006.

8. James K. Lim, interview with author, December 1, 2006.

9. Carl J. Malanga, interview with author, November 14, 2006.

10. Louise Wojcik, interview with author, November 3, 2006.

9. The National Scene

1. *The West Virginia Pharmacist* (1961), 14 [12]: 3.

2. J.L. Hayman, *The West Virginia Pharmacist* (1955), 8 [1]: 12.

3. *The West Virginia Pharmacist* (1955), 8 [6]: 6-7.

4. Anon. "Roy Bird Cook Collection Published by the University," *The West Virginia Pharmacist* (1965), 18 [1]: 4.

5. J.L. Hayman. The Medalist as a Pharmacist and Board Secretary. *The West Virginia Pharmacist* (1956), 8 [1]: 10-26.

6. Ohio Board of Pharmacy, personal communication, April 19, 2007

7. "Dr. Cook Honored by Legislature," *West Virginia Pharmacist* (1962), 15 [2]: 9-10.

8. Interview with author with American Pharmacists Association, June 27, 2005.

9. Anon. *"Fifty Years in Review."The West Virginia Pharmacist* (1955), 8[5]: 10.

10. N.W. Stewart, *Journal of the American Pharmaceutical Association* (1954), 15 [10]: 609-613.

11. *The Dominion Post* (Morgantown, W.Va.), June 3, 1955.

12. American Pharmaceutical Association News Release, January 21, 1992.

13. G.B. Griffenhagen, "150 Years of Caring: a Pictorial History of The American Pharmaceutical Association" (2002), 299.

14. Visiting Committee Records, courtesy of Mrs. J. Piper, WVU School of Pharmacy.

15. American Pharmaceutical Association, unsigned communication, November 4, 2005.

16. Curriculum vitae of Tom Menighan, April 13, 2005.

17. John Plummer, "Remarks from the 1983-1984 NABP President" from the 79th annual Meeting, held May 14-18, 1984.

18. John Plummer, President's address at the NABP 80th annual meeting held April 29-May 3, 1984.

19. *Wall Street Journal,* Thursday October 4, 2007, page D6, "FDA May Ease Prescription Drug Rules," by Jennifer C. Doreen

10. The Local and Regional Scene

1. *Kremers and Urdan's History of Pharmacy*, Glenn Sonnedecker, ed., (Philadelhia :J.P. Lippincott, 1976), 379.

2. Paul Logsdon, director of Alumni Affairs at Ohio Northern University, interview with author, February 2, 2006.

3. Anon. "Fifty Years in Review, Part 1," *The West Virginia Pharmacist* (1956), 9 [3]: 4

4. Anon. "Fifty Years in Review, Part 2," *The West Virginia Pharmacist* (1956), 9 [4]: 4 -20.

5. Obituary of Alfred Walker, *Braxton Citizens News*, April 4, 1932.

6. "West Virginia PH.A. Urges Creation of Pharmacy Department for State University," *The Pharmaceutical Era*, July 29, 1909: 99.

7. George D. Beal, presenting at the APhA General Session in Cincinnati, August 1959.

8. Anon. "Fifty Years in Review, Part 3," *The West Virginia Pharmacist* (1956), 9[5]: 6-12.

9. Ernst Stieb, *History of the American College of Apothecaries. The First Quarter Century, 1940-1965* (Washington, D.C.: American College of Apothecaries, 1970).

10. "Letter to Past Presidents," V. Hertzog, from the minutes for the Past Presidents Club, August 10, 1987.

11. V. Hertzog, minutes, August 16, 1955.

12. R.B. Cook, Past Presidents Club comments, August 16, 1955.

13. Ibid.

14. Average salary for that era provided by the National Community Pharmacists Association, April 20, 2005.

15. Mrs. J.P. Plummer, interview with author, March 24, 2005.

16. H.R. Ridenous, Past Presidents Club comments, September 20, 1964.

17. C.H. Traubert, Past Presidents Club comments, September 20, 1964.

18. J.B. Dorsey, Past Presidents Club comments, September 20, 1964.

19. Carroll Martin, interview with author, March 30, 2005.

20. Mrs. A.B. Smith, interview with author, March 30, 2005.

21. John "Jack" Neale, interview with author, March 31, 2005.

22. Martha Hickman, interview with author, March 31, 2005.

23. W. Phillips, interview with author, March 24, 2005.

24. "William J. Dixon Resigns as Secretary-Manager," *The West Virginia Pharmacist* (1965), 17 [8]: 7.

25. V. Hertzog, minutes, July 19, 1965.

26. C.E. Furbee, Jr., "The President's Message," *The West Virginia Pharmacist* (1965), 18[8]: 20.

27. "Association Pledges," *The West Virginia Pharmacist* (1965), 18[8]: 20.

28. V. Hertzog, minutes, July 15, 1968.

29. V. Hertzog, minutes, July 7, 1969.

11. WVPA Awards

1. Lee Anderson and Gregory J. Higby, *The Spirit of Voluntarism: A Legacy of Commitment and Contribution: The United States Pharmacopeia, 1820-1995* (Rockville, Md.: United States Pharmacopeial Convention, 1995).

2. "Meet Your Association Officers," *The West Virginia Pharmacist* (1965), 18 [10]: 19.

3. "Stevens Heads District Pharmacy Association," *The West Virginia Pharmacist* (1965), 18 [10]: 22.

4. Obituary of Bev Davis, *The Register-Herald* (Beckley), February 12, 2000.

5. W. Ernest Turner, interview with author, July 15, 2005.

6. "Turner Recipient of 1988 Bowl of Hygeia Award," *The West Virginia Pharmacist* (1988), 12 [3]: 7.

7. Charles V. Selby, Jr. , interview with author, March 18, 2006.

8. Carol Ann Hudachek, interview with author, June 15, 2006.

9. Lora L. Good, interview with author, June 21, 2006.

10. Lee Ann Welch, "Founder of the Fruth Pharmacy Chain Dies at 77," *Herald Dispatch* (Huntington), July 21, 2005.

11. Ibid.

12. Tim Maloney, "Fruth Got Promise from Governor on U.S. 35," *Point Pleasant Register,* July 27, 2005.

13. Obituary of Jack E. Fruth, *Point Pleasant Register*, July 27, 2005.

14. Ibid.

15. Obituary of Jack E. Fruth, *Herald Dispatch* (Huntington), December 27, 2005.

16. Obituary of Jack E. Fruth, *Point Pleasant Register*, July 21, 2005.

17. Sen. Charles C. Lanham, letter to author, June 7, 2006.

18. Thomas Menighan, interview with author, April 22, 2005.

19. "Crawford is First Recipient of Practice Excellence Award," APhA news release, January 21, 1992.

20. Sandra Justice, interview with author, July 13, 2005.

12. *Women as Leaders in the Profession*

1. Dan Rider, interview with author, February 8, 2007

2. Charles D. Chico, interview with author, July 24, 2006

3. Mary Angotti, interview with author, April 24, 2007

4. Charles D. Chico, Interview with author, July 24, 2006

5. Silvester Dinardi, Interview with author, June 23, 2006

6. Buddy Quertinmont, interview with author, July 13, 2006

7. Marie Abate, interview with author, January 25, 2007.

8. Virginia Scott, interview with author, February 12, 2006

9. Elizabeth J. Scharman, interview with author, February 12, 2006
10. Carol Hudachek, interview with author, February 7, 2007
11. Patty Johnston, interview with author, February 8, 2007
12. Sandra Justice, interview with author, February 9, 2007
13. Susan Meredith, interview with author, February 12, 2007
14. Lydia Main, interview with author, February 14, 2007
15. Karen Reed, interview with author, February 14, 2007
16. Barbara Dietz Smith, interview with author, February 12, 2007
17. Michele Vigneault McNeill, interview with author, March 16, 2007
18. Felice Joseph, interview with author, March 16, 2007
19. Edna Thaxton Buergler, interview with author, April 27, 2007

13. *Changing Roles and Responsibilities*

1. Michael E. Cunningham, interview with author, November 2, 2003
2. Judie Charlton, interview with author, October 17, 2005
3. Jimmie Mangus, interview with author, October 19, 2005
4. Robert J. Beto, interview with author, February 26, 2007
5. Brian Gallagher, interview with author, February 26, 2007
6. Stephen Brooks, interview with author, September 27, 2006
7. Karen E. Kahle, interview with author, October 5, 2006
8. Andrea Miller, interview with author, October 17, 2006
9. James Coleman, interview with author, October 3, 2006
10. John F. Cooper-Martin, interview with author, October 3, 2006
11. Michael Krupa, interview with author, October, 19, 2005
12. Curriculum vitae of Frank Lilly, dated 1990
13. Anon. Phi Lambda Upsilon Alumni. Http://www.chem.edu/plu/Alumni. htm
14. Anon. A Professor Faces a Tough, Visible, and Thankless Job. *Chronicle of Higher Education*, August 12, 1987.
15. Julie Johnson, Strong Opinions with No Apologies. *New York Times*, May 25, 1988, A22.
16. Richard Berke, citing Larry Kramer in "Ex-Leader in Gay Group Chosen for AIDS Panel," *New York Times*, July 21, 1987.
17. Richard Berke, Ex-Leader in Gay Group Chosen for AIDS Panel. *New York Times*, July 21, 1987.
18. Philip M. Boffey, "AIDS Panelist Vote to Expand Anti-Bias Law," *New York Times*, June 18, 1988.
19. Dominick P. Purpura, memorandum to the Einstein Community, July 23, 1987.

194

20. Sandra G. Boodman, "First Meeting of AIDS Panel on Rocky Path," *Washington Post*, September 10, 1987.

21. Thomas Moran, "Members of AIDS Panel Say Politics Will Not Taint Their Report," *New York Times*, September 3, 1987, B3.

22. Sandra G. Boodman, "Top Officers of AIDS Panel Step Down Over Infighting; Chairman Told Officials He Was Undermined," *Washington Post*, October 8, 1987.

23. Philip MM. Boffey, "Panel on AIDS Turns Voices of Criticism into Songs of Praise," *New York Times*, March 7, 1988.

24. Lynn Rosellini, "The Metamorphosis of the AIDS Admiral," *U.S. News and World Report,* July 4, 1988.

25. Jim Detjen, "Little Chance Polio Vaccine Trials in 1957 Started AIDS, Panel Finds," *Toronto Star*, November 1, 1992.

26. David B. Dunlap, "Frank Lilly, a Geneticist, 65. Member of National AIDS Panel" (obituary), *New York Times*, October 19, 1995.

27. Anna Marie Calcagno, interview with author, September 19, 2006.

28. Paula Jo Stout, interview with author, April 25, 2007.

29. Alice K. Pau, interview with author, December 6, 2006.

30. Valerie Schmidt Mondelli, interview with author, September 19, 2006.

31. Jan Burks Skelton, interview with author, September 19, 2006.

32. Thomas E. Menighan, interview with author, September 19, 2006.

33. Curriculum vitae of Thomas E. Menighan, dated 2005.

34. Michele Vigneault McNeill, interview with author, November 15, 2006.

Afterword. Concluding Thoughts

1. RB Steward, "The future of pharmacy: Armageddon or Pollyanna?" *The Annals of Pharmacotherapy* (1995), 29: 1292-1296

Pharmacists as Mayors

Name:	*Fred Clay Allen*	
Birth/Death:	1888 – 1969	
Education:	Ph.G., Valparaiso University College of Pharmacy, IN	1909
Pharmacy/ Practice History:	Owner, Royal Drug Store	1909 – 1969
City Served as Mayor:	Marlinton, WV	1928 – 1932
Service as State Senator:	Senator, 10th WV Senatorial District	1937 – 1956
Military Service:	Served in France (World War I) with the 80th Infantry Division in the Somme Offensive and the battles of the Meuse-Argonne	
Notable Facts:	President, WVPA	1935 – 1936
	Member, Democratic Executive Committee	1938 – 1969
	State Democratic Party Chairman	1957 – 1960
	Member, West Virginia Board of Pharmacy	1960 – 1967
	Recipient, Dr. James H. Beal Award	1955
	Honorary President, NABP	1958

Name:	*Sterling Elwood Bare, Jr.*	
Birth/Death:	1926 – 1998	
Education:	B.S., WVU College of Pharmacy	1948
Pharmacy/ Practice History:	Owner, P.A. George Rexall Pharmacy*	1948 – 1996
City Served as Mayor:	Ronceverte, WV	1963 – 1964
Civic Club Service:	Member, Ronceverte Chamber of Commerce Member and Past President, Ronceverte Rotary Club	
Notable Facts:	Served as Ronceverte City Commissioner Served on Ronceverte Police Commission.	

*Name of the pharmacy was that of previous owner, Powhatan Alexander George, who died in 1938.

Name:	*Charles William Blissitt*	
Birth/Death:	1932 –	
Education:	B.S., Southern College of Pharmacy, (Now Mercer University Southern School of Pharmacy)	
	Ph.D., University of Florida	1958
Pharmacy/ Practice History:	Assistant Professor, WVU School of Pharmacy	1958 – 1964
	Dean, St. Louis University School of Pharmacy	1964 – 1970
	Dean, University of Oklahoma College of Pharmacy	1970 – 1977
City Served as Mayor:	Morgantown, WV	1962 – 1964
City Council Service:	Chair, Morgantown Council Finance Committee Member, Building and Zoning Committee Liaison, City Council – Parking Authority	
Honors:	Rho Chi Honor Society Sigma Xi Gamma Sigma Epsilon Phi Sigma	
Notable Facts:	In 1964, at age 31, he accepted an appointment as Dean of the St. Louis University College of Pharmacy.	

Name:	*Alfonso Daniel Carolla, Jr.*	
Birth/Death:	1954 –	
Education:	B.S., WVU College of Pharmacy	1980
Pharmacy/ Practice History:	Citizens Drug Store, Welch, WV	1980 – 1981
	Owner, Bradshaw Pharmacy, Bradshaw, WV	1981 – 2004
	Staff Pharmacist, Bradshaw Rite Aid Pharmacy	2004 –
City Served as Mayor:	Bradshaw, WV	1989 – 1991
City Council Service:	Bradshaw City Council	1987 – 1989
	Bradshaw City Council	2005 – present

Name:	*Benjamin Harry Carson*	
Birth/Death:	1931 – 1994	
Education:	B.S., WVU College of Pharmacy	1954
Pharmacy/ Practice History:	Owner, College Drug Store	1956 – 1994
City Served as Mayor:	Montgomery, WV	1992 – 1994
City Council Service:	Montgomery City Council	1986 – 1992
Community Service:	Chaired Montgomery City Planning Commission President, Montgomery Business and Professional Association	
Civic Club Membership:	Past President, Montgomery Rotary Club	
Military Service:	Served to rank of First Lieutenant, USAR	1954 – 1956
Notable Facts:	Mayor Carson died of lung cancer during his second term in office on November 6, 1994.	

Name:	*William Sidney Coleman*	
Birth/Death:	1902 – 1989	
Education:	B.S., Medical College of Virginia (now Virginia Commonwealth University) School of Pharmacy	1925
Pharmacy/ Practice History:	Rose's Drug Store, Hinton, WV	1925 – 1929
	Meadow River Lumber Co., Rainelle, WV	1929 – 1931
	Owner, Coleman's Pharmacy, Lewisburg WV	1931 – 1989
City Served as Mayor:	Lewisburg, WV (Six terms as mayor)	1961 – 1973
City Council Service:	Five terms on Lewisburg City Council	1951 – 1961
Notable Facts:	President, WVPA	1938 – 1939
	First in family to become a pharmacist Nine family members followed his lead to provide 351 years of pharmacy service to West Virginia Two sons are pharmacists	

Name:	*Carl E. Furbee, Jr.*	
Birth/Death:	1924 – 1998	
Education:	B.S., WVU College of Pharmacy	1951
Pharmacy/ Practice History:	Staff pharmacist Furbee's Pharmacy Owner, Furbee's Pharmacy	1951 – 1970 1970 – 1988
City Served as Mayor:	Bridgeport, WV (six terms as mayor)	1973 – 1975 1989 – 1997
Military Service:	U.S. Army, Pacific Theater of Operations in World War II	
Honors/Awards:	WVU College of Pharmacy Outstanding Alumnus Award	1967
	Bowl of Hygeia Award	1974
	Michael Benedum Fellow Community Service Award	
Notable Facts:	President, WVPA	1965 – 1966
	Defeated for reelection after first term as mayor	1975
	Doubled city's tax base during second tenure as mayor	1989 – 1997
	Annexed site of FBI Fingerprint Division	
	Annexed Bridgeport Airport	
	Annexed land for future site for United Hospital Center	
	Annexed land for Briarwood Subdivision	
	Instrumental in development of South Hills and Shearwood subdivisions	

Name:	*Samuel George Kapourales*	
Birth/Death:	1935 –	
Education:	B.S. Chemistry, University of Richmond	1953
	B.S. Medical College of Virginia (now Virginia Commonwealth University) School of Pharmacy	1960
Pharmacy/ Practice History:	Williamson, WV	
City Served as Mayor:	Williamson, WV (ten terms as Mayor)	1979 – 1999
Notable Facts:	Member, West Virginia Board of Pharmacy	1980 – 2000*
	Reappointed to Board of Pharmacy	2005 –
	*Served on WV Board of Pharmacy	1980 – 2000
	*Served on WV Board of Pharmacy	2005 – Present
	Has owned pharmacies in WV, KY, and TN	
	Serves on Board of WV Health Care Authority	

Name:	George Karos	
Birth/Death:	1931 –	
Education:	B.S., Medical College of Virginia (now Virginia Commonwealth University) School of Pharmacy	1959
Pharmacy/ Practice History:	Owner, Patterson's Drug Store	1959 – present
City Served as Mayor:	Martinsburg, West Virginia	2000 – present
City Council Service:	Served as Martinsburg Councilman-at-large	
Notable Facts:	Director, Downtown Martinsburg Association Chairman, Martinsburg Fire Facility Committee President, Martinsburg Chamber of Commerce Member, Berkeley County Development Authority Member, Berkeley County Board of Health Berkeley County War Memorial Park President, West Virginia Board of Pharmacy Member, American Pharmacists Association Member, WV Pharmacists Association Member, Eastern Panhandle Academy of Pharmacy Honorary Alumnus, WVU School of Pharmacy Paul Harris Fellow Award, Martinsburg Rotary Club Bowl of Hygeia Award Sam Walton Business Leadership Award Distinguished Citizenship Award, Grand Lodge of Elks USA Who's Who in West Virginia Business	

Name:	Lydia DeBoni Main	
Birth/Death:	1929 –	
Education:	WVU Pre-medicine Program	1947 – 1949
	Morgantown Business College	1950
	B.S., WVU College of Pharmacy	1956
Pharmacy/ Practice History:	Owner, Main Pharmacy	1957 – present
City Served as Mayor:	Masontown, WV	1973 – 1997, 1999 – present
Memberships:	National Association of Boards of Pharmacy National Community Pharmacists Association Tri-County Council for the Boy Scouts of America Director, Preston and Tucker County Counties Health Associations	

Sustaining member, WVPA
Lions International Club

Elective Offices:	Vice President, WV Board of Pharmacy for 20 years.
	President, WVU School of Pharmacy
	Alumni Association 1992 – 1993
	President, Board of Directors, Preston and Tucker Counties
	Health Association
	Two term President of the Valley District Lions Club

Notable Facts: Task Force of Internet Pharmacy of the NABP
Chair of the Combined Advisory Group for the Vocational
   School and the Academic Center of Preston County.

Name: *William Jefferson Plyburn*

Birth/Death: 1934 – 1997

Education: Marshall University (no degree)
B.S., University of Cincinnati School of Pharmacy   1955

**Pharmacy/
Practice History:** Owner, Plyburn Village Pharmacy   1962 – 1990

**City Served as
Mayor:** Barboursville, WV   1989 – 1993

Community Service: Mayor Plyburn worked actively with the American Red
Cross, Boy Scouts of America, and sponsored both Little
League baseball and football teams

Civic Club Service: Past President Barboursville Lion's Club
Charter Member Barboursville Chamber of Commerce

Notable Facts: Barboursville Parks and Recreation Board
Barboursville Council for Retarded Children
Member, Friends of the Library
Pharmacy Consultant, Barboursville State Mental Hospital
WVPA Board of Directors

Name:	*George Bowers Rice*	
Birth/Death:	1916 – 2000	
Education:	B.A., Education, Fairmont State College	1938
	B.S., WVU College of Pharmacy	1946
Pharmacy/ Practice History:	Owner, Johnson Drug Store	1943 – 1984
City Served as Mayor:	Shinnston, WV	1962 – 1966
Honors/Awards	Outstanding Community Service Award, American Druggist	1945
	Outstanding Community Service Award, Shinnston Business and Professional Club	1945

Name:	*Emerson Van Romig*	
Birth/Death:	1876 – 1969	
Education:	Ph.G., Scio College of Pharmacy,	1899
	Ph.G., Pittsburgh College of Pharmacy,	1902
Pharmacy/ Practice History:	Owner, Romig's Drug Store Keyser, WV	1899 – 1969
	Worked in the pharmacy business office or as a greeter until his death at age 93	
City Council Service:	Served on the Keyser City Council	1909 – 1921
City Served as Mayor:	Keyser, WV	1921 – 1925
Civic Club Membership:	Charter member of Keyser Rotary Club	
	President of Keyser Rotary Club	
Notable Facts:	Charter member, WVPA	
	President, WVPA	1928
	Noted for selfless acts of kindness: When a competitor died during the depression, he sent a pharmacist to keep the pharmacy open until the widow could sell the store.	
	At the height of the 1918 flu epidemic, he passed kidney stones. Despite excruciating pain, he continued to fill prescriptions and did not miss a single day during the epidemic.	

Name:	*Richard Emerson Romig*	
Birth/Death:	1918 – 1983	
Education:	B.S., WVU College of Pharmacy	1942
Pharmacy/ Practice History:	Owner, Romig's Drug Store, Keyser, WV	1946 – 1983
City Served as Mayor:	Keyser, WV	1956 – 1961
Service Club Membership:	Keyser Rotary Club	
Military Service:	Served in the U.S. Army Air Corps during World War II as a pilot at Lackland Field, San Antonio, Texas	
Notable Facts:	Mineral County Board of Education	1940s – 1950s
	Mineral County United Fund Steering Committee	

Name:	*Donald Chatham Sinclair*	
Birth/Death:	1927 – 1999	
Education:	B.A., Political Science, West Virginia University	1953
	B.A., Economics, West Virginia University	1953
	B.S., WVU College of Pharmacy	1957
	M.A., Bible Philosophy, American Bible Institute	
Pharmacy/ Practice History:	Owner, Sinclair's Pharmacy	1962 – 1999
City Council Service:	Served nine consecutive terms as Bethlehem City councilman	1973 – 1991
City Served as Mayor:	Bethlehem, WV (4 consecutive terms as mayor)	1991 – 1999
Military Service:	U.S. Naval Air Corps (Air-Sea Rescue) during World War II	
Community Service:	Served on Wheeling Urban Renewal Authority	
	Known locally for his drug-abuse prevention programs	
Civic Club Service:	President, Wheeling Kiwanis Club	
	Member, Wheeling Junior Chamber of Commerce	
Elective Office:	Past President, Ohio/Marshall County Pharmaceutical Association	
	Vice President, WVU School of Pharmacy Alumni Association	1963
	President, WVU School of Pharmacy Alumni Association	1967

204

Name:	*Newell Williamson Stewart*	
Birth/Death:	1900 – 1989	
Education:	Ph.G., Department of Pharmacy, WVU School of Medicine	1923
Pharmacy/ Practice History:	J. H. Bean Drug Co, Moundsville, WV	1923 – 1926
	Retail pharmacy, Phoenix, AZ	1926 – 1952
City Served as Mayor:	Phoenix, AZ	1942 – 1944
Professional Office Held:	President, Arizona Pharmaceutical Association	1936
	President, APhA	1955
	Executive VP, National Pharmaceutical Council	1954 – 1965
	Secretary, Arizona Pharmaceutical Association	1941
	Secretary, Arizona Pharmaceutical Association	1943 – 1954
	Secretary, Arizona Pharmaceutical Association	1968 – 1971
	Secretary, Arizona Board of Pharmacy	1937
	Secretary, Arizona Board of Pharmacy	1940 – 1952
Notable Facts:	Presidential Appointment to the War Man Power Commission during World War II	
	Led effort to establish a Department of Pharmacy in the College of Liberal Arts, University of Arizona	1947
	Instrumental in establishing the College of Pharmacy at the University of Arizona	
	Founder, Arizona Pharmacy Historical Foundation	1977
	Interim Exec. Secretary, AZ Pharmaceutical Association	1968
Honors:	Outstanding Alumnus Award, WVU College of Pharmacy	1953
	Honorary President, AZ Community Pharmacist Association	1980
	Honorary President, ASHP	1980
	Doctor of Science (Hon.) degree, AZ College of Pharmacy	1956

Name:	*James Lawrence Turner*	
Birth/Death:	1928 – 1982	
Education:	B.S., WVU College of Pharmacy	1950
	M.S. Biochemistry, West Virginia University	1964
	Ph.D. Biochemistry, West Virginia University	1976

Pharmacy/
Practice History:	Staff pharmacist, Malone's Deep Cut	
	Rate Drugs	1950 – 1952
	Staff pharmacist, Troxell's Pharmacy	1952 – 1958
	Owner, Turner's Pharmacy	1958 – 1982

City Council
Service:	Fairmont, WV	1977 – 1979

City Served
as Mayor:	Fairmont, WV	1979 – 1982

Notable Facts:	Faculty, Department of Chemistry,	
	Fairmont State College (FSC)	
	(now Fairmont State University)	1967 – 1982
	Developed a biochemistry program for FSC	1965
	Served on the Pharmacy and Therapeutics Committee of the West Virginia Board of Health	
	Member, National Association of Advisors to the Health Professions	
	Member, Board of Directors of the Union Mission of Fairmont	
	Member, Fairmont United Way Allocations Committee	
	Member, Fairmont Community Council	

Behind the Counter to the Front Lines

Name:	*Ralph Raymond Ferguson*	
Birth/Death:	1920 – 1944	
Education:	B.S., WVU College of Pharmacy	1943
Military Service:	U.S. Army (European Theatre of Operations)	1943 – 1944
	Participated in Normandy D-Day Invasion	1944
Highest Rank Held:	Second Lieutenant	
Honors/Awards:	Purple Heart Medal (posthumous)	1944
	European Theatre of Operations Ribbon with one Bronze Service Star	1944

Name:	*James William Fredlock*	
Birth/Death	1929 –	
Education:	B.S., WVU College of Pharmacy	1951
	Associate Infantry Company Officers Course	1951
Military Service:	179th Infantry Regiment, 45th Division (Korea)	1951 – 1953
Highest Rank Held:	Captain, Infantry	
Honors/Awards:	Bronze Star Medal	1953
	Combat Infantry Badge	1952
	Korean Service Medal	1953
	United Nations Korean Service Medal	1953
	Republic of Korea Korean War Medal	1953
Pharmacy Practice:	Staff Pharmacist, Fredlock's Pharmacy, Morgantown, WV	1953 – 1970
	Owner, Fredlock's Pharmacy, Morgantown, WV	1970 – 1986
	Owner, Chestnut Ridge Pharmacy, Morgantown, WV	1986 – 1987
	Owner, Bruceton Pharmacy, Bruceton Mills, WV	1985 – 1990

Name:	*Douglas Dennis Glover*	
Birth/Death:	1929 –	

Education:	B.S., WVU College of Pharmacy	1951
	Associate Infantry Company Officers Course	1951
	Medical Field Service School	1952
	B.S. Medicine, WVU School of Medicine	1959
	Doctor of Medicine,	
	Emory University School of Medicine	1961
	Residency in Obstetrics and Gynecology,	
	Grady Memorial Hospital, Atlanta, GA	1961 – 1965

Military Service:	U.S. Army (Korea)	1951 – 1953

Highest Rank Held:	First Lieutenant (USAR)	1952

Academic Appointments:	Associate Professor,	
	Marshall University School of Medicine	1982 – 1987
	Professor, Ob/Gyn, Marshall University	
	School of Medicine	1987
	Professor, Ob/Gyn, WVU School of Medicine	1987 – 2004
	Professor Emeritus, WVU School of Medicine	2004 – Present

Offices Held:	President, Marion County (WV)	
	Pharmaceutical Association	1956
	President, WVU School of Pharmacy Alumni	
	Association	1978 – 1979
	President, Southern WV Pharmacists	
	Association	1984 – 1985
	President, Monongalia County (WV) Medical Society	1991
	U.S.P. General Committee of Revision	1990 – 2005
	Chair, Ob/Gyn Advisory Panel, USPC	1990 – 2000
	Vice President, Mon Valley Pharmacists	
	Association	1989
	Treasurer, WVU School of Pharmacy Alumni Association	1994 – Prese

Military Awards:	Bronze Star Medal	1953
	Purple Heart Medal	1953
	Combat Medical Badge	1952
	Expert Infantry Badge	1951
	Korean Service Medal with three Bronze	
	Service Stars	1953
	United Nations Korean Service Medal	1953
	National Defense Service Medal	1953
	Republic of Korea Korean War Medal	1953

Honors/Awards:	Pete Royal Memorial Award for Outstanding	
	Professional and Community Service (Georgia)	1981
	WVU School of Pharmacy Outstanding Alumnus Award	1982
	WVU School of Pharmacy Outstanding Service	
	Award	1972, 1987
	WVPA Dr. James H. Beal Award	1989
	Outstanding Service to the Armed Forces of the	
	United States Award	1997
	Phi Lambda Sigma Leadership Honorary	1997
	WVU School of Pharmacy Distinguished Alumnus	
	Award	1999
	Who's Who in America, 56th – 62nd Editions	2001 – 2008
	WVU Most Loyal Faculty Mountaineer Award	2004
	WVU School of Medicine	
	Faculty Recognition Award	1997, 2002, 2005
	WVU School of Medicine Dean's Award for Excellence	2005

Pharmacy	Staff Pharmacist, Corbett's Drug Store,	
Practice:	Romney, WV	1953 – 1954
	Staff Pharmacist, H-H Drug Co., Fairmont, WV	1954 – 1957

Medical Practice: Senior Partner, Ob/Gyn Affiliates, Marietta, GA   1965 – 1982

Name:	*John Joseph "Jack" Halki*	
Birth/Death:	1926 – 2000	
Education:	WVU, College of Arts and Sciences (no degree)	1946 – 1947
	B.S., WVU College of Pharmacy	1947 – 1950
	WVU Graduate School (no degree)	1952
	B.S., WVU School of Medicine	1954
	Doctor of Medicine, Medical College of Virginia	1956
	Residency in Ob/Gyn, Medical College of Virginia	1960
	Ph.D. Pharmacology, University of Kansas	1963
	Brook AFB, Texas: Primary Course in	
	Aerospace Medicine	1963
Military	U.S. Navy: Seaman/Pharmacist Mate,	
Service:	Commander of an LCM landing craft,	1944 – 1946
	USAF Medical Corps/Flight Surgeon	
	Consultant to the USAF Surgeon General	1957 – 1981
Highest Rank		
Held:	Brigadier General, USAF Medical Corps	1981

Academic Appointments:	Assistant Clinical Professor of Ob/Gyn, University of Texas Health Sciences Center at San Antonio	1968 – 1970
	Associate Clinical Professor of Ob/Gyn, University of Texas Health Sciences Center at San Antonio	1970 – 1975
	Associate Clinical Professor of Ob/Gyn, Wright State University School of Medicine	1976 – 1980
	Associate Professor of Ob/Gyn, Wright State University School of Medicine	1980 – 1987
	Professor of Ob/Gyn, Wright State University School of Medicine	1987 – 1989
	Professor of Pharmacology and Toxicology, Wright State University School of Medicine	1987 – 1989
	Professor Emeritus, Wright State University	1989 – 1999
Honors/Awards:	American Campaign Medal	1945
	Asia-Pacific Campaign Medal with one Service Star	1945 – 1946
	World War II Victory Medal	1946
	Rho Chi Pharmacy Honor Society	1949
	The Merck Award	1950
	National Defense Medal	1957, 1959
	Air Force Outstanding Unit Award with two Oak Leaf Clusters	1965, 1975
	Air Force Commendation Medal	1965
	Legion of Merit 1976, 1979	
	Distinguished Service Medal	1981
	American Academy of Family Physicians Teaching Award	1982
	Nicholas J. Thompson Distinguished Professorship of Obstetrics and Gynecology	1985
	Outstanding Alumnus Award, WVU School of Pharmacy	1986
	Alpha Omega Alpha Honorary (Faculty)	1987 – 1999
	Kermit Krantz Air Force Award, Armed Forces District, ACOG	1988
	Who's Who in America	1988

Name:	*Leo Harry Knowlton*	
Birth/Death:	1927 –	
Education:	B.S., WVU College of Pharmacy	1952
Military Service:	U.S. Marine Corps	1944 – 1946
	U.S. Navy	1947 – 1947
	U.S. Marine Corps Reserve	1947 – 1952
	U.S. Marine Corps	1950 – 1951
Military Campaigns:	Wonsan, Hungnam, Chosan	1950
Highest Rank Held:	Sergeant	
Honors/Awards:	World War II Victory Medal	1946
	National Defense Service Medal	1952
	Korean Service Medal	1952
	Republic of Korea Korean War Medal	1953
	United Nations Korean Service Medal	1953
Pharmacy Practice:	Temple Drug Store, Nitro, WV	1952 – 1956
	Miller Drug Store, Dunbar, WV	1956 – 1972
	Staff Pharmacist, Charleston Memorial Hospital	1972 – 1978
	Staff Pharmacist, Charleston General Hospital	1978 – 1987

Name:	*John Patrick Plummer*	
Birth/Death:	1919 – 2004	
Education:	B.S., WVU College of Pharmacy	1943
Military Service:	U.S. Navy, Pacific Theatre of Operations, World War II	1943 – 1946
Highest Rank Held:	Commander, U.S.N.R	1973
Honors/Awards:	WVU School of Pharmacy Outstanding Service Award	1956, 1960
	WVU School of Pharmacy Outstanding Alumnus Award	1961
	WVPA Dr. James Hartley Beal Award	1987
	WVPA Outstanding Pharmacist Award	1957, 1966
Notable Facts:	Member, City of Fairmont Planning Committee	
	Member, Board of Directors, Fairmont General Hospital	
	Served five terms as president of parochial school board	

Pharmacy Practice:	Staff Pharmacist, Bonn's Prescription Shop,	
	Fairmont, WV	1950 – 1955
	Staff Pharmacist/Owner, H - H Drug Company	1955 – 1989
	Member, National NABP Executive Committee	1978
	President, WVU School of Pharmacy	
	Alumni Association	1961
	Member, WV State Board of Pharmacy	1967 – 1986
	President, WV Pharmacists Association	1964 – 1965
	Treasurer, NABP Executive Committee	1978
	National President, NABP	1983 – 1984
	Adjunct Professor Clinical Pharmacy, WVU	

Name: *Michael Alfonso Rafferty*

Birth/Death: 1903 – 1944

Education:	Ph.C., WVU College of Pharmacy, Morgantown, WV	1929
	Ph.D., Biochemistry, Duquesne University,	
	Pittsburgh, PA	1931
	Ph.D., Pharmacology, Duquesne University,	
	Pittsburgh, PA	1931
	B.S., WVU School of Medicine, Morgantown, WV	1933
	Doctor of Medicine, Rush Medical College, Chicago, IL	1935
	Residency in Medicine Rush Medical College,	
	Chicago, IL	1937

Military Service: U.S. Army Medical Corps   1942 – 1944

Highest Rank Held: Major   1944

Honors/Awards:	Lehn and Fink Gold Medal	1929
	Purple Heart Medal (posthumous)	1944

Medical Practice:	Faculty, WVU School of Medicine,	
	Morgantown, WV	1937 – 1941
	Research, Miles Laboratories, Elkhart, IN	1941 – 1942

Name: *Clyde Eugene Reed*

Birth/Death: 1922 –

Education:	B.S., WVU College of Pharmacy	1951
	Doctor of Dental Surgery,	
	University of Maryland Dental School	1957

| Military Service: | U.S. Army, Pacific Theatre of Operations | 1942 – 1946 |

Military Service:	U.S. Army, Pacific Theatre of Operations	1942 – 1946
Military Honors/ Awards:	Asiatic Pacific Campaign Medal with 2	
	Bronze Service Stars	1946
	American Defense Service Medal	1946
	Good Conduct Medal	1946
	World War II Victory Medal	1946
	Combat Infantry Badge	1944
Highest rank:	T-4	
Dentistry Practice:	Baltimore, Maryland	1957 – 1987

Name:	*Edward William Rockis*	
Birth/Death:	1928 – 1988	
Education:	B.S., WVU College of Pharmacy	1951
	Associate Infantry Company Officers Course	1952
	MTC 0605-0600 Course, Ft. Benning, Georgia	1952
Military Service:	U.S. Army (Korea)	1951 – 1953
Highest Rank Held:	First Lieutenant	
Honors/Awards:	Purple Heart Medal	1952
	Combat Infantry Badge	1952
	Purple Heart with Oak Leaf Cluster	1953
	Silver Star Medal	1953
	Korean Service Medal with two Bronze	
	Service Stars	1953
	United Nations Korean Service Medal	1953
	National Defense Service Medal	1953
	Meritorious Service Medal of Greek	
	Expeditionary Forces in Korea	1954
Pharmacy Practice:	Pharmacist/Owner, City Pharmacy, Morgantown, WV	1954 – 1988
Notable Facts:	President, WVU School of Pharmacy	
	Alumni Association	1971
	WVU School of Pharmacy Outstanding Alumni Award	1975
	WVU School of Pharmacy Outstanding Service Award	1985

Name:	*Ralph Stuart Stevenson*	
Birth/Death:	1923 –	
Education:	B.S., WVU College of Pharmacy	1951
Military Service:	USAF, European Theatre of Operations	1943 – 1945
	Prisoner of War	1944 – 1945
	101st Airborne Infantry Division	1951 – 1952
Highest Rank Held:	Staff Sergeant (World War II)	
	First Lieutenant (Korean War)	
Military Honors/ Awards:	Purple Heart Medal	1945
	Two Presidential Unit Commendations	1945
	Air Medal with 4 Oak Leaf Clusters	1945
	European Theatre Medal with 3 Bronze Service Stars	1945
	National Defense Medal	1952
	Good Conduct Medal	1945
	World War II Victory Medal	1945
Pharmacy Practice:	Staff Pharmacist, Marlinton, WV	1953 – 1957
	Staff Pharmacist, Hinton, Oak Hill, Keystone, WV	1957 – 1959
	Pharmacist/Manager, Concord, North Carolina	1959 – 1987
	Relief Pharmacist, Concord, North Carolina	1987 – 1995

Deans of the West Virginia
University School of Pharmacy
(in order of service)

Name:	*J. Lester Hayman*	
Year Born/Year Death:	1896 – 1963	
Education:	Ph.C., University of Michigan College of Pharmacy	1919
	B.S., University of Michigan College of Pharmacy	1919
	M.Sc., University of Michigan College of Pharmacy	1925
Pharmacy Practice:	Summers in West Virginia	1922
Age named Dean:	42	
Honor Societies:	Rho Chi Honor Society	
	Alpha Chi Sigma	
	Phi Lambda Upsilon	
	Phi Sigma Biological Society	
Notable Facts:	First recipient, Dr. James H. Beal Award	1947
	President, American Association of Colleges of Pharmacy	1948 – 1949
	President and Secretary, National Conference of Pharmaceutical Association Secretaries	
	Second Vice President, American Pharmaceutical Association	
	Chair, three major APhA committees	
	President, WVPA	1959 – 1960
	Member, USP Committee of Revision	1930 – 1950
	Delegate to United States Pharmacopeial Convention from WVU School of Pharmacy	1930 – 1960

Name:	*Raphael O. Bachmann, Ph.D.*	
Year Born/Year Death:	1921 – 1972	
Education:	B.S. Pharmaceutical Chemistry,	
	Creighton University	1942
	Ph.D. Pharmaceutical Chemistry,	
	Purdue University	1950
Military Service:	Communications Officer, U.S. Navy,	
	served to rank of Lieutenant Junior Grade	1944 – 1946
Pharmacy Practice:	No record	
Age named Dean:	40	
Honor Societies:	Rho Chi Honor Society	
	Sigma Xi	
	Phi Lambda Upsilon	
	Alpha Sigma Nu	
	Alpha Chi Sigma	
	Kappa Phi	
Notable Facts:	President, American Association of	
	Colleges of Pharmacy	1969 – 1970
	Regional Director, American Board of	
	Diplomats in Pharmacy	
	Director, American Foundation for Pharmaceutical	
	Education	
	Fellow, American Foundation for Pharmaceutical	
	Education	
	Director, West Virginia Pharmacists Association	

Name:	*Louis A. Luzzi, Ph.D.*	
Year Born/Year Death:	1932 – 2007	
Education:	B.S., University of Rhode Island	1959
	M.S., University of Rhode Island	1962
	Ph.D. Pharmaceutics, University of Rhode Island	1966
Pharmacy Practice:	Assistant Professor, University of Georgia	1966
	Associate Professor, University of Georgia	1969
	Professor, University of Georgia	1973
Age Named Dean:	41	

Honor Societies:	Sigma Xi
	Rho Chi Honor Society
	Phi Sigma
	Phi Kappa Phi

Notable Facts:	Fellow of American Academy of Science

Consultantships:	Food and Drug Administration, State of West Virginia
	(Finance and Administration Department)
	Veterinary Corporation of America
	Abbott Laboratories
	Hoffman LaRoche
	Sandoz Pharmaceuticals
	William S. Merrell Laboratories
	Mylan Laboratories
	A. H. Robbins Company
	Eurand, Incorporated

Name:	*Sidney A. Rosenbluth, Ph.D.*	
Year Born/Year Death:	1933 –	
Education:	B.S., University of Oklahoma School of Pharmacy	1955
	Residency in Hospital Pharmacy, University of	
	Arkansas Medical Center	1961
	M.S., University of Texas at Austin	1962
	Ph.D. Pharmaceutics/Biochemistry, University of	
	Texas at Austin	1966
	Postdoctoral Research Fellowship, Bath University,	
	Bristol, U.K.	1966
Pharmacy Practice:	University of Tennessee at Austin	1966 – 1973
	Professor of Pharmaceutics/Director	
	of Pharmacy	1973 – 1981
	Director of Pharmacy Affairs,	
	City of Memphis Hospital	1973 – 1981
	Director of Pharmacy Affairs,	
	West Tennessee Chest Hospital	1973 – 1981
	Director of Pharmacy Affairs,	
	Tennessee Psychiatric Institute	1973 – 1981
Age Named Dean:	48	
Notable Facts:	Scholar in Residence, AACP	1994 – 1995
	Best Rho Chi Chapter Advisor (honored twice)	

Name:	*George Robert Spratto, Ph.D.*	
Year Born/Year Death:	1940 –	

Education:	B.S. Fordham University College of Pharmacy	1961
	University of Wisconsin, Department of Pharmacology	1961 – 1962
	Ph.D. in Pharmacology, University of Minnesota	1966

Pharmacy Practice:	FDA, Bureau of Drug Abuse Control and Bureau of Narcotics and Dangerous Drugs	1966 – 1968
	Assistant Professor, Purdue University	1968 – 1971
	Associate Professor, Purdue University	1971 – 1979
	Professor of Pharmacology and Pharmacal Sciences	1979 – 1995
	Associate Dean for Professional Programs, Purdue University School of Pharmacy	1984 – 1995
	Dean, West Virginia University School of Pharmacy	1995 – 2006
	Interim Director, Mary Babb Randolph Cancer Center, WVU School of Medicine	2000 – 2001

Age Named Dean: 55

Honoraries:
Sigma Xi
Rho Chi Honor Society
Kappa Epsilon (honorary member)
Kappa Psi
Omicron Delta Kappa
Iron Key (Purdue University President's Honorary)
Phi Delta Chi
Phi Kappa Phi
Phi Lambda Sigma

Notable Facts:
Purdue University: Henry Heine Award for Outstanding Teaching
Amoco Foundation Outstanding Undergraduate Teaching Award
American School Health Association Distinguished Service Award
Merck Sharp and Dohme Award for Outstanding Achievement In the Profession of Pharmacy
M. Beverley Stone Award for Non-Academic Advising
U.S. Department of Defense Seven Seals Award, Operation Desert Storm

West Virginia Novartis Pharmacy Leadership Award
West Virginia Society of Health System Pharmacists
   Schwartz Pharma Leadership Award
National Association of Chain Drug Stores Award
Member, Accreditation Council for Pharmacy
   Education   2004 – Present
President, Accreditation Council for
   Pharmacy Education   2006 – Present

Name: *Patricia A. Chase, Ph.D.*

Year Born/Year Death: 1948 –

Education:

B.S., Albany College of Pharmacy	1971
ASHP Residency in Hospital Pharmacy	1971 – 1972
M.S. in Hospital Pharmacy, University of North Carolina	1985
Wharton School of Business, LDI Fellow	1993
Ph.D. in Administration, University of Colorado	1995
College Management Program, Carnegie Mellon University, H. John Heinz III School of Public Policy and Management, Pittsburgh, PA	1997

Pharmacy Practice:

Staff Pharmacist, Plaza Pharmacy, Houlton, Maine	1972 – 1973
Director of Pharmacy Services, Houlton Regional Hospital, Houlton, Maine	1973 – 1983
Clinical Pharmacist, Moses Cone Hospital, Greensboro, North Carolina	1983 – 1985
Assistant Director for Administrative Services, Pharmacy Department, Monteflore Medical Center	1985 – 1986
Associate Professor, University of Oklahoma College of Pharmacy/Director of Pharmacy Oklahoma Medica Center Hospital	1986 – 1990
Professor of Pharmacy, School of Pharmacy, University of Colorado HSC, Denver, CO	1990 - 1996
Assistant/Associate Dean, College of Pharmacy, Western University of Health Sciences, Pomona, CA	1997 – 2000
Professor and Dean, College of Pharmacy and Health Sciences Center, Butler University, Indianapolis, IN	2000 – 2006

Gates Wigner Professor and Dean,
    WVU School of Pharmacy   2006 – Present
Age named Dean: 57

Honoraries: Phi Lambda Sigma National Leadership Society
Rho Chi Honor Society
Kappa Delta Phi International Honor Society for
    Education

Notable Facts: Honorary Member of Maine Society of Hospital
    Pharmacists

The National Scene: West Virginians as Presidents of the APhA and the NABP

Name:	*Roy Bird Cook, L.L.D. (Hon.)*	
Birth/Death	1886 – 1961	
Education:	Graduate, Weston High School	1904
	Apprenticeship with Minter B. Ralston in Weston from age 13 to 19	
	Doctor of Law (Hon.), West Virginia University	1938
Pharmacy Practice:	Joined West Virginia Pharmaceutical Association	1911
	Community Practice, Huntington, WV	1909 – 1919
	Partnership with Othor O. Older, Charleston, WV	1926 – 1944
	Community Practice, Charleston, WV	1944 – 1961
Notable Facts:	President, WVPA	1918
	Secretary, WVPA	1923 – 1926
	President, NABP	1938 – 1939
	President, American Pharmaceutical Association	1942 – 1943
	Member, Board of Pharmacy	1925
	Secretary, Board of Pharmacy	1932 – 1961
	Dr. James H. Beal Award, WVPA	1947
	Remington Medal, APhA	1955
	Posthumously recognized by WV State Legislature as champion of pharmaceutical ethics, recipient of the Remington Honor Medal, and for achieving national recognition as an historical author	1962

Name:	*Newell Williamson Stewart*	
Birth/Death	1900 – 1989	
Education:	Ph.G., West Virginia University College of Pharmacy	1923
Military Service:	U.S. Army, A.E.F., World War I (France)	1918 – 1919
Pharmacy Practice:	Community pharmacy practice, Moundsville, WV	1923 – 1926
	Pharmacy Owner, Phoenix, AZ	1926 – 1952
Notable Facts:	Secretary Arizona Board of Pharmacy	1937 – 1952
	Editor, *Arizona Pharmacist*	1947 – 1954
	President, National Association of Boards of Pharmacy	1948 – 1949
	Executive Vice President, National Pharmaceutical Council	1954 – 1965
	President, American Pharmaceutical Association	1955
	Chair, Phoenix War Loan Drive, World War II	1943 – 1946
	Chair, Phoenix (AZ) Community Chest	
	Board of Trustees, Phoenix (AZ) Memorial Hospital	
	Outstanding Alumnus, WVU College of Pharmacy Alumni Association	1953
	Mayor of Phoenix, Arizona	1942 – 1944

Name:	*Thomas Edward Menighan*	
Birth/Death:	1952 –	
Education:	B.S. in Pharmacy (Cum Laude), West Virginia University School of Pharmacy	1974
	M.B.A., Averett College, APhA Community Pharmacy Management Program, University of North Carolina	
Pharmacy Practice:	Chain Store Pharmacy, Zanesville, Ohio,	1974 – 1976
	Chain Store Manager, Danville, Virginia	1976 – 1978
	Owner, Medicine Shoppe Pharmacy, Huntington, WV	1978 – 1998
	Formed Option Care Home Infusion Services for WV, KY, OH	1981
	President, American Pharmacists Association	1987 – 1988
	Vice President, Operations Pharmark Corp	1992 – 1993
	President & CEO, SymRx, Inc., Rockville, MD	2000 – 2005

Notable Facts:	Bowl of Hygeia award	1984
	NARD Pharmacy Leadership Award	1985
	WVU School of Pharmacy Preceptor of the Year Award	1986
	WVU School of Pharmacy Outstanding Alumnus Award	1987
	Dr. James Hartley Beal Award, WVPA	1999
	WVPA/Merck Outstanding Achievement in	
	Profession of Pharmacy award	1995

Name: *John Patrick Plummer*

See Appendix B, Behind the Counter to the Front Lines

Name: *David Steven Crawford*

See Appendix E, Sixty-Ninth President of WVPA

The Local and Regional Scene
Presidents of WVPA

*Every effort was made by the author to provide a full accounting of the career of each of the presidents of the West Virginia Pharmacists Association. However, in some cases, such information was unavailable.

Name:	*Stephen Alfred Walker,* First President	
Birth/Death:	1863 – 1932	
Education:	Northwestern Ohio Normal School (now Ohio Northern University)	
	Apprenticeship at two Ohio pharmacies	
Pharmacy Practice:	Registered in WV	1892
	Owner, Juergens & Walker, Sutton, WV	1901 – 1932
Notable Facts:	President, WVPA	1906 – 1907
	Appointed to the West Virginia Board of Commissioners of Pharmacy by	
	Governor A.B. White	1901 – 1932
	Secretary, Board of Pharmacy	1902 – 1932

Name:	*Ed Bruce Dawson,* Second President	
Birth/Death:	Unknown – 1946	
Education:	Unknown	
Pharmacy Practice:	Registered in WV	1899
	Wheeling, WV	1899 – 1925
	Cleveland, Ohio	1925 – 1946
Notable Facts:	President, WVPA	1907 – 1908
	Vice President, WVPA	1906 – 1907

Name:	*Arch Kreig,* Third President	
Birth/Death:	1868 – 1953	
Education:	Ph.G. degree, Cincinnati College of Pharmacy	1889
Pharmacy Practice:	Cincinnati and Belaire, Ohio	1889 – 1896
	Registered in WV	1896
	Pharmacy Practice, Charleston, WV	1896 – 1915
	Kreig, Wallace & McQuaide Company, Charleston, WV	1915 – 1926
	Kreig Drug Company, Charleston, WV	1926 – ?
	Trivillians Drug Store, Charleston, WV	? – 1953
Notable Facts:	President, WVPA	1908 – 1909
	Gold Medal, Highest Academic Standing in Pharmacy Class	1889
	First elected Secretary, WVPA (2 year term)	1906 – 1908
	Re-elected Secretary, WVPA (served 36 years)	1911 – 1947
	Honorary Life Member, WVPA	1947

Name:	*William W. Irwin,* Fourth President	
Birth/Death:	Unknown – 1924	
Education:	Unknown	
Pharmacy Practice:	Registered in WV	1883
	Community Practice, Wheeling, WV	?
Notable Facts:	President, WVPA	1909 – 1910
	President, Wheeling Retail Druggists Association	
	Sheriff, Ohio County, WV	
	Postmaster, Wheeling, WV	

Name:	*William Samson Vinson,* Fifth President
Birth/Death:	1868 – 1948
Education:	Marshall College, Huntington, WV (no degree)
	Dunsmore Business College, Staunton, VA (no degree)
	Apprenticeship with T. N. Boggess, Huntington, WV

Pharmacy Practice:	Registered in West Virginia	1896
	Owner, Fountain Drug Store,	
	Huntington, WV	1896 – 1926
	Founder and President,	
	Huntington Wholesale Drug Company	
	(later the Huntington Division of	
	McKeson and Robbins)	1926 – 1933
Notable Facts:	First Treasurer, WVPA	1906 – 1909
	President, WVPA	1910 – 1911
	Founder NARD	
	One of founders, WVPA	

Name:	*George Orville Young,* Sixth President	1911 – 1912
Birth/Death:	1873 – 1958	
Education:	Ph.G. degree, Scio College, Scio, Ohio	1896
Pharmacy Practice:	Cumberland, Maryland	1896 – 1900
	Sales Representative,	
	Wm. S. Merrell Company	1900 – 1902
	Pharmacy Owner, Buckhannon, WV	1902 – 1946
Notable Facts:	Secretary, WVPA (2 Year Term)	1909 – 1911
	President, WVPA	1911 – 1912
	Founding member, WVPA	1906
	Founder, American Druggists' Fire	
	Insurance Co.	1906
	Vice President, American Druggists'	
	Insurance Company	1906 – 1926
	Member, Board of Directors, American	
	Druggists' Insurance Company	1912 – 1958
	Founder, Central National Bank of	
	Buckhannon, (now Chase Bank)	1932
	WV State Senate	1935 – 1947
	Founder, WV State Chamber of Commerce	1936
	Minority Leader, West Virginia State Senate	1941, 1943
	First Chairman, WV Game and Fish Commission	?
	Honorary President, APhA	1958
	Author of several critically acclaimed books	
	Dr. James H. Beal Award	

Name:	*Walter C. Price,* Seventh President	
Birth/Death:	1877 – 1941	
Education:	Apprenticeship in Ohio	
Pharmacy Practice:	Registered in West Virginia	1898
	Staff Pharmacist, Kreig & Price,	
	Charleston, WV	1898 – 1913
	Staff Pharmacist, Huntington Drug	
	Company, Huntington, WV	1913 – 1941
Notable Facts:	President, WVPA	1912 – 1913
	Postmaster, Huntington, WV	1928
	Founder, Huntington Rotary Club	
	Sponsored a bill prohibiting sale of liquor	
	in West Virginia pharmacies	1913

Name:	*Walter E. Dittmeyer,* Eighth President	
Birth/Death:	1879 – 1937	
Education:	West Virginia University (no degree)	1900 – 1902
	Ph.G., Philadelphia College of Pharmacy	1904
Pharmacy Practice:	Registered in West Virginia	1904
	Community Practice, Harpers Ferry, WV	1904 – 1937
Notable Facts:	President, WVPA	1913 – 1914
	Vice President, WVPA	1910 – 1911

Name:	*John R. Elson,* Ninth President	
Birth/Death:	1880 – 1950	
Education:	Wheeling Business College	1900
	Ph.G., Scio College of Pharmacy	1902
Pharmacy Practice:	Registered in WV	1903
	Pharmacy Owner, WV	1904 – 1922
	Practiced Pharmacy, North Carolina	1931 – 1950
Notable Facts:	President, WVPA	1914 – 1915
	First Vice President, WVPA	1913 – 1914
	Member, WV House of Delegates	1912 – ?
	Member, WV State Board of Pharmacy	1917 – 1922

Name:	*Bert E. Downs,* Tenth President	
Birth/Death:	1879 – Unknown	
Education:	Apprenticeship in Greenup, KY	
	Graduated Ohio Northern College	1902
Practice of Pharmacy:	Pharmacy Practice, Cattletsburg, KY	1902 – 1903
	Owner, Welch, WV	1904 – ?
Notable Facts:	President, WVPA	1915 – 1916
	Secretary, WVPA	1914 – 1915
	Member, WV State Board of Pharmacy	1911 – 1923

Name:	*C. A. Neptune,* Eleventh President	
Birth/Death:	1879 – 1955	
Education:	Apprenticeship with W. I. Boreman	1893 – 1904
Pharmacy Practice:	O.J. Stout and Company, Parkersburg, WV	1904 – 1945
Notable Facts:	President, WVPA	1916 – 1917
	Secretary, WVPA	1912 – 1914
	Life Member (Hon.), WVPA	1946
	Member, WVPA Legislative Committee	
	Instrumental in establishing the WVU College of Pharmacy	
	Instrumental in enacting the West Virginia narcotic law, one of the nation's first	

Name:	*Othor O. Older,* Twelfth President	
Birth/Death:	1872 – 1963	
Education:	Morris Harvey College (now University of Charleston), Charleston, WV	?
	Ph.B. degree, Cincinnati College of Pharmacy	1901
Pharmacy Practice:	Owner, Browning and Older Drug Company	1901 – 1902
	Owner, Older Drug Company	1902 – 1926
	Owner, Older-Cook Drug Company	1926 – 1944
	Owner, Older Drug Company	1944 – 1950
Notable Facts:	President, WVPA	1917 – 1918
	Member, WV State Board of Pharmacy	1920 – 1925
	Vice President, NARD	1941

Name:	*Roy Bird Cook,* Thirteenth President	
Birth/Death:	1886 – 1961	
Education:	Apprenticeship with Minter B. Ralston	1899 – 1905

Practice of Pharmacy:	Registered in WV	1905
	Employee, Ralston and Bare, Weston, WV	1905 – 1907
	Owner, Ralston and Cook, Drug Store, Weston, WV	1907 – 1909
	Owner, Frederick Pharmacy, Huntington, WV	1909 – 1919
	Owner, Kreig, Wallace and McQuaid Company, Charleston, WV	1919 – 1926
	Owner, Older-Cook Drug Company, Charleston, WV	1926 – 1944
	Owner, Cook Drug Company, Charleston, WV	1944 – 1961

Notable Facts:	President, WVPA	1918 – 1919
	President, APhA	1935 – 1936
	Secretary-Treasurer, WVPA	1923 – 1926
	Member, WV Board of Pharmacy	1925 – 1956
	Secretary, WV Board of Pharmacy	1932 – 1956
	President, NABP	1938 – 1939
	Honorary LLD degree, West Virginia University	1938
	Dr. James H. Beal Award	1949
	APhA's Remington Medal	1955
	Life Member, WVPA	1951

Name:	*John C. Davis,* Fourteenth President	
Birth/Death:	1875 – Unknown	
Parents:	Unknown	
Education:	Unknown	
Pharmacy Practice:	Registered in WV	1914
	Associate, Hoge-Davis Drug Company	1914 – 1921
Notable Facts:	President, WVPA	1919 – 1920

Name:	*Ivan S. Davis,* Fifteenth President	
	President, WVPA	1920 – 1921
	No additional information available	

Name:	*F. C. Kramer,* Sixteenth President	
	President, WVPA	1921 – 1922
	No additional information available	

Name:	*J. Charles Hall,* Seventeenth President	
	President, WVPA	1922 – 1923
	No additional information available	

Name:	*Fred B. Watkins,* Eighteenth President	
Birth/Death:	1888 – 1963	
Education:	Unknown	
Practice:	Owner, Grafton Drug and Chemical Co.	1907 – 1933
Notable Facts:	President, WVPA	1923 – 1924
	Member, WV House of Delegates	1923 – 1924
	Member, WV House of Delegates	1931 – 1932
	State Fire Marshal	1933 – 1943
	Clerk, State Senate	1943 – 1945
	State Beer Commissioner	1945 – 1947
	Past President, Grafton Rotary Club	
	Past President, West Virginia Rexall Clubs	

Name:	*Powhatan Alexander George,* Nineteenth President	
Birth/Death:	1863 – 1938	
Education:	Ohio Northern University (Aida, Ohio)	1896
Practice:	Owner, George's Rexall Drug Store, Ronceverte, WV (one of the earliest Rexall Drug Stores in West Virginia, perhaps in the Nation).	1904 – 1940s
Notable Facts:	President, WVPA	1924 – 1925
	Former mayor of Ronceverte	

Name:	*Gaylord "Gay" Hess Dent,* Twentieth President	
Birth/Death:	1885 – 1951	
Education:	Ph.G., Western University of Pennsylvania (now University of Pittsburgh)	1908
Military Service:	Member, WV National Guard	
Practice:	Pharmacist and Manager, McVicker's Drug Store, Morgantown, WV	1906 – 1951
Notable Facts:	President, WVPA	1925 – 1926
	Treasurer, Salvation Army	
	Member, Morgantown Masonic Bodies	
	Member, Sons of American Revolution	
	Charter Member, Morgantown Kiwanis Club	
	Member, The Odd Fellows	

Name:	*H. C. Wallace,* Twenty-First President	
	President, WVPA,	1926 – 1927
	No additional Information available	

Name:	*Emerson Van Romig,* Twenty-Second President	
Birth/Death:	1875 – 1969	
Education:	Ph.G., Scio College of Pharmacy	1899
	Ph.G., Pittsburgh College of Pharmacy	1902
Pharmacy Practice:	Thomas, WV and Elkins, WV	1899 – 1903
	Owner, Romig Drug Company, Keyser, WV	1903 – 1969
Notable Facts:	Charter Member, WVPA	1906
	President, WVPA	1928 – 1929
	Mayor, Keyser, WV	1921 – 1925
	Member, Keyser City Council	1909 – 1921
	Charter Member, Keyser Rotary Club	1922 – 1923
	President, Keyser Rotary Club	1922 – 1923
	Founding Director, National Bank of Keyser	1933 – 1965
	President, Mineral County Board of Education	1942 – 1945

Name:	*S. M. Bledsoe,* Twenty-Third President
	President, WVPA 1928 – 1929
	No additional information available

Name:	*Earl L. Fortney,* Twenty-Fourth President
Notable Facts:	President, WVPA 1929 - 1930
	No additional information available

Name:	*Charles H. "Dan" Goodykoontz,* Twenty-Fifth President
Birth/Death:	1881 – 1943
Education:	University of Maryland College of Pharmacy 1902
Pharmacy Practice:	Bluefield, WV and Bristol, VA 1902 – 1907
	Founded Goodykoontz Drug Company, Bluefield, WV 1907
Military Service:	Unknown
Notable Facts:	President, WVPA 1930 – 1931
	Founder, Goodykoontz Drug Company
	Founded, East End Pharmacy 1923
	Founded, Fairview Pharmacy Unknown

Name:	*Ernest Kenworthy Hoge,* Twenty-Sixth President
Birth/Death:	1871 – 1969
Education:	Ph.G., Scio College of Pharmacy
Military Service:	None
Pharmacy Practice:	Owner, several Pharmacies in the Wheeling WV ?– 1969 area. Mr. Hoge practiced pharmacy in Wheeling until his death at age 97. At the time of his death he was the oldest practicing pharmacist in the state
Notable Facts:	President, WVPA 1931 – 1932
	Dr. James H. Beal Award 1953
	Centennial Pharmacist of Year 1963
	Honorary President of Past Presidents Club 1966

Name:	*William Reed Crane,* Twenty-Seventh President	
Birth/Death:	1870 - 1937	
Education:	Unknown	
Military Service:	None	
Pharmacy Practice:	Fairmont, WV	1906 – 1936
Notable Facts:	President, WVPA	1932 – 1933

Name:	*Charles Vinton Selby,* Twenty-Eighth President	
Birth/Death:	1903 – 1972	
Education:	Ph.G., Louisville College of Pharmacy	1924
Military Service:	None	
Pharmacy Practice:	Selby's Drug Store, Clarksburg, WV	1925 – 1954
	Schwab's Drug Store, Kingwood (post retirement)	1955 – 1972
Notable Facts:	President, WVPA	1933 – 1934
	First Secretary-Treasurer, American College of Apothecaries	1940 – 1950
	Treasurer, American College of Apothecaries	1950 – 1964
	Treasurer Emeritus, American College of Apothecaries	1964 – 1972
	American Board of Diplomats	
	Honorary Alumnus, WVU School of Pharmacy	

Name:	*Fred Clay Allen,* Twenty-Ninth President	
Birth/Death:	1888 – 1969	
Education:	Ph.G. degree, Valparaiso University College of Pharmacy	1909
Military Service:	U.S. Army, World War I	
Practice of Pharmacy:	Owner, Royal Drug Store, Marlinton, WV	1922 – 1963
Notable Facts:	President, WVPA	1934 – 1935
	WV Board of Pharmacy	1933 – 1969
	Honorary President, NABP	1958
	Dr. James Hartley Beal Award	1955
	Member, WV State Senate	1936 – 1956

President Pro Tempore, WV Senate	1945, 1949, 1951	
	1953, 1955	
Mayor, Marlinton, WV	1928 – 1932	
Member, Pocahontas County Democratic Executive Committee	1938 – 1969	

Name: *Robert Reginald Pierce,* Thirtieth President

Birth/Death: 1889 – 1965

Education: University of Maryland School of Pharmacy   1912

Military Service: None

Pharmacy Practice: Community pharmacy, Thomas, WV   1912 – 1921
Owner, Pierce Pharmacy, Morgantown, WV   1921 – 1962

Notable Facts: President, WVPA,   1935 – 1936
Honorary Alumnus, WVU School of Pharmacy   ?
    WVPA

Name: *Emmett Oswald Wiseman,* Thirty-First President

Birth/Death: 1903 – 1989

Education: Ph.G., Louisville College of Pharmacy   1925

Military Service: None

Pharmacy Practice: Owner, Wiseman Drug Company, Fayetteville, WV

Notable Facts: President, WVPA   1937 – 1938
First Vice President, WVPA   1936 – 1937
Second Vice President, WVPA   1935 – 1936
Third Vice President, WVPA   1934 – 1935
Secretary-Treasurer, American College of Apothecaries
Charter Member, American College of Apothecaries
Past President, Central WV Academy of Pharmacists
President, Fayette County Board of
    Education   1963 – 1967
Member, Fayette County Commission
Member, Fayette Rotary Club
Fifty-year member of Masonic Lodge (Shriner)
Honorary Alumnus, WVU School of Pharmacy
Member, WV House of Delegates
Member, WV State Senate Member
Member, State Board of Health

Name:	*Granville S. Flesher,* Thirty-Second President	
	President, WVPA	1937 – 1938

No additional information available

Name:	*William Sidney Coleman,* Thirty-Third President	
Birth/Death:	1902 – 1989	
Education:	B.S., Medical College of Virginia (now part of Virginia Commonwealth University) School of Pharmacy	1925
Military Service:	None	
Pharmacy Practice:	Roses' Drug Store, Rainelle, WV	1925 – 1927
	Meadow River Lumber Company, Rainelle, WV	1927 – 1929
	Coleman's Pharmacy, Lewisburg, WV	1929 – 1989
Notable Facts:	Joined WVPA a year before graduating from pharmacy school	1924
	First of nine pharmacists in his extended family	
	Two sons have also served as WVPA Presidents	
	President, WVPA	1938 – 1939
	Member, Lewisburg City Council	1951 – 1961
	Mayor, Lewisburg, WV	1961 – 1973
	Bowl of Hygeia Award	1966
	President Past Presidents Club	1967
	Dr. James Hartley Beal Award	1975

Name:	*F. A. McFarlin,* Thirty-Fourth President	
	President, WVPA	1939 – 1940

No additional information available

Name:	*Rodney A. Barb,* Thirty-Fifth President	
	President, WVPA	1940 – 1941

No additional information available

Name:	*Carl Walker,* Thirty-Sixth President	
	President, WVPA	1941 – 1942

No additional information available

Name:	*Lynn Lionel Carson,* Thirty-Seventh President
Birth/Death:	1893 – 1969
Education:	Unknown
Military Service:	Unknown
Pharmacy Practice:	Carson and Scott Drug Store, Wellsburg WV

Notable Facts:

President, WVPA	1942 – 1943
First Vice President, WVPA	1941 – 1942
Second Vice President, WVPA	1939 – 1940
Honorary Alumnus, WVU School of Pharmacy	
Director, Wellsburg National Bank	
Director, Advanced Federal Savings & Loan Ass'n	
Director, Steubenville Ohio Valley Hospital	
Past Master, Wellsburg Masonic Lodge (33rd degree)	

Name:	*Harry A. Goodykoontz,* Thirty-Eighth President
Birth/Death:	1891 – 1951
Education:	Apprenticeship, possibly under his brother
Military Service:	Unknown
Pharmacy Practice:	Bluefield, WV

Notable Facts:

President, WVPA	1943 – 1944
First Vice President, WVPA	1942 – 1943
Second Vice President, WVPA	1941 – 1942
Member, WVPA Council	1946 – 1949

Name:	*L. C. Harlan,* Thirty-Ninth President
	President, WVPA 1945 – 1946

No additional information available

Name:	*James A. Patterson,* Fortieth President
	President, WVPA 1946 – 1947

No additional information available

Name:	*Edgar B. Moore,* Forty-First President	
Birth/Death:	Unknown	
Pharmacy Practice:	Clarksburg, WV	
Notable Facts:	President, WVPA	1944 – 1945
	Third Vice President, WVPA	1943 – 1944
	Second Vice President, WVPA	1944 – 1946
	First Vice President, WVPA	1946 – 1947
	Member, State Board of Health	1965 – 1973
	Bowl of Hygeia Award	1964
	James H. Beal Honor Award	1965
	President, Past Presidents of WVPA Club	1968

Name:	*Virgil Ross Hertzog,* Forty-Second President	
Birth/Death:	1896 – 1998	
Education:	Ph.G., WVU College of Pharmacy	1922
Military Service:	Served in AEF (France), U.S. Army,	
	World War I	1918 – 1919
	Commander, "40/8" Veterans Organization	
Pharmacy Practice:	Owner, Worthington Pharmacy,	
	Worthington, WV	1925 – 1970
Notable Facts:	President, WVPA (first WVU graduate)	1949 – 1950
	President, WVU College of Pharmacy	
	Alumni Association	1950 – 1951
	First Vice President, WVPA	1947 – 1948
	American Druggist Citation for Outstanding	
	Community Service	1950
	WVU College of Pharmacy Outstanding	
	Alumnus Award	1954
	Dr. James Hartley Beal Award	1977
	WVU College of Pharmacy Outstanding	
	Service Award	1970
	Bowl of Hygeia Award	1975
	Third Vice President, WVPA	1944 – 1945
	Secretary, Past Presidents Club	1966 – 1969
	Oldest practicing pharmacist in West Virginia	

Name:	*Albert Kiddy Walker,* Forty-Third President	
Birth/Death:	1896 – 1962	
Education:	Ph.G., WVU College of Pharmacy	1922
Military Service:	Pilot, U.S. Army Air Corps, World War I	
Pharmacy Practice:	Owner, Walker's Drug Store, Sutton, WV	?
Notable Facts:	President, WVPA	1949 – 1950
	First Vice President, WVPA	1948 – 1949
	Second Vice President, WVPA	1947 – 1948
	Third Vice President, WVPA	1946 – 1947

Name:	*Clyde N. Roberts,* Forty-Fourth President	
Birth/Death:	1905 – 1997	
Education:	Ph.C., Cincinnati College of Pharmacy	1928
Military Service:	None	
Pharmacy Practice:	Lawrence Drug Store, Huntington WV	1942 – 1997
Notable Facts:	President, WVPA	1950 – 1951
	First Vice President, WVPA	1949 – 1950
	Second Vice President, WVPA	1948 – 1949
	Third Vice President, WVPA	1947 – 1948
	Dr. James Hartley Beal Award	1963
	WVU School of Pharmacy Honorary Alumnus	
	Member, WV State Board of Pharmacy	1957 – 1961

Name:	*J. B. Dorsey,* Forty-Fifth President	
Birth/Death:	1896 – 1967	
Education:	WVU (no degree)	1919 – 1920
Military Service:	U.S. Army, World War I	1918 – 1919
Pharmacy Practice:	Passed licensure exam	1923
	Operated the J.B. Dorsey Drug Company in Moundsville, WV	1923 – 1967
Notable Facts:	President, WVPA	1951 – 1952

Name:	*Edgar Dale Tetrick,* Forty-Sixth President	
Birth/Death:	1914 – 1970	
Education:	B.S., WVU College of Pharmacy	1940
Military Service:	None	
Pharmacy Practice:	Owner, Tetrick's Pharmacy, Shinnston, WV	1940 – 1970
Notable Facts:	Third Vice President, WVPA	1949 – 1950
	Second Vice President, WVPA	1950 – 1951
	First Vice President, WVPA	1951 – 1952
	President, Shinnston Area Development Association	
	Member, West Virginia State Board of Pharmacy	1958 – 1963
	Officer, WV Pilots Association	
	32nd Mason, Scottish Rite Bodies	

Name:	*Harry Alan Goodykoontz, Jr.,* Forty-Seventh President	
Birth/Death:	1924 – Unknown	
Education:	B.S., WVU College of Pharmacy	1948
Military Service:	Private, US Army	1943 – 1945
Pharmacy Practice:	Registered in West Virginia	1948
	Community pharmacy, Bluefield, WV	1948 – 1974
	St. Lukes Hospital Pharmacy, Bluefield, WV	1974 – 1981
	Bluefield Regional Medical Center	1981 – 1990
Notable Facts:	President, WVPA	1952 – 1953
	First Vice President, WVPA	1951 – 1952
	Member, WVPA Council	1952 – 1955
	Past President, Southern Appalachian Pharmaceutical Association	
	Director, Flat Top National Bank	1964 –

Name:	*William B. Stuck, Jr.,* Forty-Eighth President	
Birth/Death:	1905 – 1989	
Education:	Ph.G., West Virginia University College of Pharmacy 1925	
Military Service:	U.S. Coast Guard, World War II	
Highest Rank Attained:	Chief Pharmacists Mate	

Pharmacy Practice: Partner, Nichols & Stuck, Charles Town, WV
Co-owner, Stuck and Alger Pharmacy, Charles
   Town, West Virginia

Notable Facts:	President, WVPA	1954 – 1955
	First Vice President, WVPA	1953 – 1954
	Second Vice President, WVPA	1953 – 1953
	Past President, WVU Pharmacy Alumni Ass'n	1952
	Member, WV Board of Pharmacy	1959 – 1969
	Past President WV Eastern Panhandle Pharmaceutical Association	
	President of Jefferson Development Corporation	1958 –

Name:	*James Ray Fredlock,* Forty-Ninth President	
Birth/Death:	1901 – 1989	
Education:	Ph.G., WVU College of Pharmacy	1927
Military Service:	None	

Pharmacy Practice:	Owner, Fredlock's Pharmacy, Morgantown, WV	1943 – 1989

Notable Facts:	President, WVU Pharmacy Alumni Association	1938 & 1954
	President, WVPA	1954 – 1955
	President, WVU Alumni Association	1959 – 1960
	President, Morgantown Chamber of Commerce	1952 – 1953
	West Virginia University Executive Council	1956
	WVU College of Pharmacy Outstanding Service Award	1954
	WVU College of Pharmacy Outstanding Alumnus Award	1959
	Board of Directors, First National Bank of Morgantown	
	Elder (30 years), First Presbyterian Church, Morgantown, WV	
	Mountain Men's Honorary	1927
	Phi Kappa Sigma Fraternity	

Name:	*Curtis George "Si" Meadows,* Fiftieth President	
Birth/Death:	1904 – 1960	
Education:	Ph.G., WVU College of Pharmacy	1923
Military Service:	None	
Pharmacy Practice:	Staff Pharmacist, Oak Hill, WV	1924 – 1928
	Partner, Aracoma Drug Company,	
	Logan, WV	1928 – 1959
Notable Facts:	President, WVPA	1956 – 1957
	First Vice President, WVPA	1955 – 1956
	Second Vice President, WVPA	1954 – 1955
	Third Vice President, WVPA	1953 – 1954
	President, Logan County Chamber of Commerce	
	Member, Logan Rotary Club	

Name:	*Charles Horner Troxell,* Fifty-First President	
Birth/Death:	1892 – 1967	
Education:	Ph.G., University of Pittsburgh	1915
Military Service:	AEF, World War I, U.S. Army	
	Medical Corps	1918 – 1919
Pharmacy Practice:	Mountain City Drug Company,	
	Fairmont, WV	1919 – 1920
	Owner, Troxell Pharmacy, Fairmont, WV	1920 – 1950
	Owner, Troxell & Turner Pharmacy,	
	Fairmont, WV	1950 – 1958
Notable Facts:	Founder, Marion County Pharmaceutical Association	
	First President, Marion County Pharmaceutical Association	
	President, WVPA	1957 – 1958
	First Vice President, WVPA	1956 – 1957
	Second Vice President, WVPA	1955 – 1956
	Third Vice President, WVPA	1954 – 1955
	Recipient: Bowl of Hygeia Award	1959
	50 Year Member Masonic Lodge	

Name:	*Harold Richard "Red" Ridenour,* Fifty-Second President
Birth/Death:	Unknown
Education:	Ph.C., WVU College of Pharmacy 1930
Military Service:	Unknown
Pharmacy Practice:	Huntington, WV
Notable Facts:	Elected Fellow of American College of Apothecaries 1958 One of the first hospital pharmacists in West Virginia

Name:	*Joseph Lester Hayman,* Fifty-Third President
	President, WVPA 1959 – 1960
	See Appendix for Deans

Name:	*Minter Bailey Ralston, Jr.,* Fifty-Fourth President
Birth/Death:	1902 – 1983
Education:	University of Maryland School of Pharmacy 1925
Military Service:	None
Pharmacy Practice:	Pharmacist, Weston State Hospital Associated in practice at various times with J. H. Bare, J.S. Lewis and Roy Bird Cook. Owner, Ralston's Pharmacy, Weston, WV 1925 – 1975

Notable Facts:	President, WVPA 1960 – 1961
	Bowl of Hygeia Award 1961
	President, 25-Year Veterans of Pharmacy Practice 1961
	Treasurer, American College of Apothecaries 1964 – 1970
	Past President, Weston Lions International
	Ralston's Pharmacy, founded in 1856, was the
	   oldest continuous-run pharmacy in WV
	Regional Director, American College of
	   Apothecaries 1963
	Member, Central (WV) Academy of Pharmacy
	32nd degree Mason. Knights Templar

Name:	*Harry Reginald Lynch,* Fifty-Fifth President	
Birth/Death:	1918 – Unknown	
Education:	B.S., WVU College of Pharmacy	1948
Military Service:	U.S. Navy, European-African-Asiatic Theaters	1942 - 1946
Highest Rank Held:	Chief Pharmacist Mate	
Pharmacy Practice:	Owner, Lynch Pharmacy, Charleston, WV	
Notable Facts:	President, WVPA	1961 – 1962
	First Vice President, WVPA	1960 – 1961
	Second Vice President, WVPA	1959 – 1960
	Third Vice President, WVPA	1958 – 1959
	Member, WVPA Council	1962 – 1965
	Consultant to WV Department of Mental Health	
	Governor's Advisory Committee on Mental Health	

Name:	*Charles Herbert Traubert,* Fifty-Sixth President	
Birth/Death:	1907 – 1987	
Education:	Ph.C., WVU College of Pharmacy	1929
	FBI National Police Academy	1943
Military Service:	None	
Pharmacy Practice:	Hoge-Davis Drug Company, Wheeling, WV	1929 – 1937
	Traubert Drug Company, Wheeling, WV	1945
	Hooverson Heights Drug Company, Follansbee, WV	
	Cove Valley Drug Company, Weirton, WV	
Notable Facts:	President, WVPA	1962 – 1963
	Secretary, West Virginia Board of Pharmacy	1960 – 1987
	Member, West Virginia Board of Pharmacy	1961 – 1987
	Dr. James H. Beal Award	1967
	NABP Distinguished Service award	1977
	WVU College of Pharmacy Outstanding Alumnus Award (only alumnus to receive award twice)	1958, 1965
	WVU School of Pharmacy Outstanding Service Award	1968
	Outstanding Dedication in the Profession of Pharmacy Award, Northern Panhandle (WV)	
	Academy of Pharmacy	1967
	West Virginia State Senate	1948 – 1960
	Follansbee WV Citizen of the Year	1969
	Sheriff, Brooke County, WV	1937 – 1944

Name:	*Joseph William Pugh, Sr.,* Fifty-Seventh President
Birth/Death:	1917 – 1994
Education:	B.S. in Pharmacy, WVU College of Pharmacy 1939
Military Service:	Pilot, Air Sea Rescue, U.S. Navy Air Corps 1942 – 1945
Pharmacy Practice:	Patterson's Drug Store, Martinsburg, WV 1939 – 1975
	Eckerd Drug Store, Martinsburg, WV 1975 – 1981
Notable Facts:	President, WVPA 1963 – 1964
	Past President, Eastern WV Academy of Pharmacy Member, WV Board of Pharmacy 1970 – 1975
	Chairman, Memorial Gifts Division, American Cancer Society
	Member, WVU College of Pharmacy Visiting Committee
	Bowl of Hygeia Award 1960

Name:	*John Patrick Plummer,* Fifty-Eighth President
Birth/Death:	1919 – 2004
Education:	B.S., WVU College of Pharmacy 1943
Military Service:	Served to rank of Lt. Commander, U.S. Navy, World War II 1943 – 1946
Pharmacy Practice:	Bonn's Prescription Shop, Fairmont, WV 1946 – 1955
	Pharmacist/Owner, H - H Drug Company Fairmont, WV 1955 – 1989
Notable Facts:	President, WVU School of Pharmacy Alumni Association 1960 – 1961
	President, West Virginia Pharmacists Association 1964 – 1965
	Recipient (twice), WVPA Outstanding Pharmacist Award ?
	Recipient, Dr. James Harvey Beal Award 1987
	WVU School of Pharmacy Outstanding Alumnus Award 1961
	Recipient (twice), WVU School of Pharmacy Outstanding Service Award 1956, 1961

Recipient, Pepsodent Award	1965
Member, WV Board of Pharmacy	1967 – 1986
Treasurer, NABP	1980 – 1981
President Elect, NABP	1982 – 1983
President, West Virginia Board of Pharmacy	1981 – 1986
President, NABP	1983 – 1984
Chairman, NABP	1984 – 1985
Member, Fairmont Planning Commission	
Board of Directors, Fairmont General Hospital	1965 – 1989

Name: *Carl Edwin Furbee, Jr.,* Fifty-Ninth President

Birth/Death: 1924 – 1998

Education: B.S., WVU College of Pharmacy   1951

Military Service: Served, U.S. Army (Infantry), Asiatic - Pacific
Theatre of Operations (New Guinea and Moratai)
World War II   1942 – 1946

Pharmacy Practice: Furbee's Pharmacy, Bridgeport, WV   1951 – 1988

Notable Facts:

Mayor (6 terms), Bridgeport, WV	1973 – 1975
	1989 – 1997
President, WVPA	1965 – 1966
President, WVU School of Pharmacy Alumni Association	1972
Recipient, WVU School of Pharmacy Outstanding Alumnus Award	1967
Recipient, Bowl of Hygeia Award	1974
Recipient, Michael Benedum Fellow Community Service Award	
Member, Legislative Committee of NARD	1966 – 1967
Board of Trustees, APhA	

Name: *John H. "Jack" Neale,* Sixtieth President

Birth/Death: 1929 –

Education: B.S., WVU College of Pharmacy   1952

Military Service: Staff Sergeant, U.S. Army, Ft. Benning, GA   1953 – 1955

Pharmacy Practice:	Practiced with Fred Allen, Marlinton, WV	1952 – 1953
	President, Neale's Drug Store, Elkins, WV	1955 – 1973
	State of WV, Health Care Benefits Unit	1970 – 1975
	Pharmacy practice, Malden, WV	1975 – 1978
	Director of Pharmacy, Hygeia Facilities Foundation	1978 – 1985
	Director of Pharmacy, Montgomery General Hospital, Montgomery, WV	1995 – 1997
	Appointed, National Association of Health Facility Licensure, a national advisory group to Medicaid and Medicare programs	
	West Virginia Nursing Home Licensing Board, (appointed by Governor Hulett Smith, reappointed by Gov. Arch Moore)	1967, 1971

Notable Facts:	President, WVPA	1966 – 1967
	Third Vice President, WVPA	1963 – 1964
	Second Vice President, WVPA	1964 – 1965
	First Vice President, WVPA	1965 – 1966
	Outstanding Businessman of the Year, Beta Alpha Beta business honorary	1958
	Board of Directors, Elkins Industrial Development Corporation	
	President, Elkins Junior Chamber of Commerce	
	President, Elkins Retail Merchants Association	
	Member (4 terms), Elkins YMCA Board of Trustees	
	Vice-President Elkins Retail Credit Association	
	Board of Directors, Randolph County United Fund	
	Member, Rotary International	
	Exulted Ruler, Elks Lodge	

Name:	*Ray L. Masterson,* Sixty-First President	
Birth/Death:	1908 – 1989	
Education:	Ph.C. degree, Ohio Northern University	1929
Military Service:	Unknown	
Pharmacy Practice:	Pharmacist, McKinely Pharmacy, Parkersburg WV	1929 – 1934
	Pharmacist, Parkersburg Central Pharmacy	1934 – 1965
	Owner, Parkersburg Central Pharmacy	1965 –
	Chief Pharmacist, Moundsville General Hospital	1975 – 1977

Notable Facts:	President, WVPA	1967 – 1968
	First Vice President	1966 – 1967
	Second Vice President, WVPA	1965 – 1966
	Third Vice President, WVPA	1964 – 1965
	Past President, Parkersburg Academy of Pharmacy	
	Instrumental in organizing Poison Control Centers at Camden-Clark and St. Joseph Hospitals Chaired a committee to revise the WVPA's Constitution and bylaws	1966
	Honorary Alumnus, WVU School of Pharmacy	1966
	Member, President's Advisory Committee, NARD	1967 – 1977?
	32nd degree Scottish Rite Mason	
	Member, Parkersburg Rotary International Club	
	Member, Nemesis Temple of the Shrine	

| Name: | *Albert Flurnoy* "Sixty" *Bond*, Sixty-Second President |
| Birth/Death: | 1900 – 1977 |

| Education: | Potomac State College (no degree) | |
| | Ph.C., WVU College of Pharmacy | 1925 – 1928 |

| Military Service: | None |

Pharmacy Practice:	Pharmacy owner, Vienna, WV	1928 – 1930
	Sales Rep/District Manager, Upjohn Company, Kalamazoo, Michigan	1930 – 1943
	Owner, Bond Drug Store, Clendenin, WV	1943 – 1951
	Gaston Drug Store, Belington, WV	1951 – 1956
	Charleston Memorial Hospital, Charleston, WV	1952 – 1953
	Bond Drug Store, Charleston, WV	1953 – 1974

Notable Facts:	President, WVPA	1968 – 1969
	First Vice-President, WVPA	1967 – 1968
	Second Vice-President, WVPA	1966 – 1967
	Third Vice-President, WVPA	1965 – 1966
	President, Kanawha Valley Pharmacy Ass'n	
	Past President, WVU School of Pharmacy Alumni Association	1965
	Recipient, Lehn and Fink Medal (First in Class)	1928
	Designed the Dept. Public Assistance Pharmacy Program for State of West Virginia that became the model for the nation	1960s

Recipient, WVU School of Pharmacy
    Outstanding Service Award   1964
Recipient, Dr. James Hartley Beal Award   1969

Name:	*Guy Nelson Lang,* Sixty-Third President	
Birth/ Death:	1924 – 1985	
Education:	B.S. in Pharmacy, WVU College of Pharmacy	1952
Military Service:	Veteran of World War II	
Pharmacy Practice:	Lang's Pharmacy, Moorefield, WV	1957 – 1985
Notable Facts:	President, WVPA	1969 – 1970
	First Vice President, WVPA	1968 – 1969
	Second Vice President, WVPA	1967 – 1968
	Third Vice President, WVPA	1966 – 1967
	Recipient: Bowl of Hygeia Award	1962
	Member West Virginia State Board of Pharmacy	1963 – 1973
	President, WV Board of Pharmacy	1970 – 1971
	President, WVU Pharmacy Alumni Association	1958
	WVU School of Pharmacy Outstanding Alumnus Award	1970
	Dr. James Hartley Beal Award	1979
	Received A.H. Robbins Award for Outstanding Community Service	1960
	WVU Pharmacy Alumni Association Outstanding Service Award	1958
	Member, Eastern West Virginia Academy of Pharmacy	
	Member, Moorefield Lion's International Club	
	Chair, Hardy County Health Board	
	Former member Moorefield Town Council	

Name:	*Robert Hugh Shirey,* Sixty-Fourth President	
Birth/Death:	1921 – 1988	
Education:	B.S. in Pharmacy, WVU College of Pharmacy	1942
Military Service:	Served to rank of Lieutenant J.G. on U.S. Navy destroyer USS Dewey in World War II	
Pharmacy Practice:	Staff Pharmacist, Beckley Drug Co.,	
	Beckley, WV	1946 – 1954
	Beckley Medical Arts Pharmacy,	1954 – 1986
Notable Facts:	President, WVPA	1970 – 1971
	Past President, New River Pharmaceutical Ass'n	
	Charter Member, WVSHP	
	Chair, WVPA Welfare Committee	
	Member, WVPA Executive Committee	
	President, Beckley Citizens' Scholarship Foundation	1969
	Beckley-Raleigh Chamber of Commerce	
	32nd degree Mason (Knights Templer)	

Name:	*William Sidney Coleman,* Sixty-Fifth President of WVPA	
Birth/Death:	1902 – 1989	
Education:	B.S., Medical College of Virginia School of Pharmacy (now Virginia Commonwealth University)	1925
Military Service:	None	
Pharmacy Practice:	Roses Drug Store, Hinton, WV	1925 – 1929
	Meadow River Lumber Company, Rainelle, WV	1929 – 1931
	Owner, Coleman's Pharmacy, Lewisburg, WV	1931 – 1989
Notable Facts:	President, WVPA	1938 – 1939
	Mayor, Lewisburg, WV	1960 – 1973
	Member, Lewisburg City Council	1951 – 1961
	Past Potentate Beni Kedm Temple	1961
	Recipient: Bowl of Hygeia Award	1966

Name:	*David Walter Miller,* Sixty-Sixth President	
Birth/Death:	1932 –	
Education:	B.S. degree in Pharmacy, WVU School of Pharmacy	1960
Military Service:	Staff Seargent, U.S.A.F.,*	1952 – 1956
Pharmacy Practice:	Staff Pharmacist, Cabell Huntington Hospital,	1960 – 1962
	Owner of pharmacies in Sistersville,	
	Paden City, and Middlebourn, WV	1965 –
Notable Facts:	President, WVPA	1972 – 1973
	Director, WVPA	1972
	Rho Chi, Kappa Psi, Phi Lambda Upsilon	
	Executive Committee, WVPA	
	Past President, Mid-Ohio Pharmacists Association	
	Director, 1st Federal Savings & Loan Association	

Name:	*Robert Browning Pierce,* Sixty-Seventh president	
Birth/Death:	1921 –	
Education:	B.S. in Pharmacy	1942
Military Service:	None *	
Pharmacy Practice:	Pierce Drug Store with his father.	1960 – 1983
	Relief pharmacist for Fredlock's Pharmacy and	
	the Oakland Maryland area.	1983 – 1995
Notable Facts:	* Employed at U.S. Rubber Co. in Detroit Michigan during World War II. He worked on a team that developed a bullet-proof fuel tank for military aircraft.	

Name:	*Jack Edward Fruth,* Sixty-Eighth President

Birth/Death:	1928 – 2005

Education:

Duke University (no degree)	1946 – 1948
B.S., The Ohio State University School of Pharmacy	1951
Master of Public Service degree (Hon), University of Rio Grande, Ohio	1986
Graduate, Dale Carnegie Course	

Pharmacy Practice:

Gallagher Drug Company, Xenia, Ohio	1951 – 1952
Founder, Owner, and CEO of Fruth Pharmacy Chain (22 stores in West Virginia and Ohio)	1952 – 2005

Notable Facts:

President, WVPA	1973 – 1974
National Chair, Affiliated Associated Drug Stores	1989 – 1990
President, Point Pleasant Chapter Rotary International	1962
President, Board of Trustees Rio Grande University	1996 – 1998
President, Point Pleasant Chapter Rotary International	1962
Recipient, Bowl of Hygeia Award	1977
Recipient, Dr. James H. Beal Award	1995
Recipient, The Ohio State University College of Pharmacy Distinguished Alumni award	1993
Recipient, WV Entrepreneur of the Year Lifetime Achievement ward	1999
Recipient, Distinguished West Virginian Award, presented by Governor Cecil Underwood	1999
U.S. Route 35 named Fruth-Lanham Highway by Governor Bob Wise	2005

Appointments:

President, Board of Trustees, Pleasant Valley Hospital	1982 – 1983
President, Mason County Chamber of Commerce	1968
Board of Directors, Green Acres Regional Center, Inc.	1960 – 1967
Director, Peoples Bank, Point Pleasant, WV	1965 – 2006
Member, West Virginia Board of Pharmacy	1992 – 2003

Name:	*David Stephen Crawford,* Sixty-Ninth President	

| **Birth/Death:** | 1945 – 2007 | |

Education:	B.S., WVU School of Pharmacy	1968
Military Service:	None	
Pharmacy Practice:	Community pharmacy practice, Elkins, WV	1968 – 2007

Notable Facts:

President, WVPA	1975 – 1976
President, Pharm-C Consultants, Elkins, WV	1975 – Present
Appointed to WV Health Advisory Committee	1975
Developed WV Health Systems Agency	1976
President, APhA Academy of Pharmacy Practice	1979 – 1980
President, WVU School of Pharmacy Alumni Association	1988 – 1989
Speaker, APhA House of Delegates	1981 – 1983
Member, WVU School of Pharmacy Visiting Committee	1975 – 1995
President, American Pharmaceutical Association	2003
Member, Review Panel, Handbook for Nonprescription Drugs	
Recipient, Squibb President's Award	1976
WVU School of Pharmacy Outstanding Alumnus	1976
Recipient, Dr. James Hartley Beal Award	1983
Recipient, Bowl of Hygeia Award	1987
Recipient, APhA Practice Excellence Award	1992

Name:	*Robert E. Hickman,* Seventieth President	

| **Birth/Death:** | Unknown | |

| **Education:** | B.S. in pharmacy, University of Cincinnati | 1962 |

| **Military Service:** | Unknown | |

| **Pharmacy Practice:** | Huntington, WV | |

Notable Facts:

President, WVPA	1976 – 1977
President, SWVP	1972
Director, WVPA	1970 – 1971
Member, WV Society Hospital Pharmacists	
Phi Eta Sigma Honorary	1959
Rho Chi Honorary	1959

Name:	*Jack Shephard Huggins,* Seventy-First President
Birth/Death:	1926 – 2006
Education:	B.A. degree in Biological Sciences, Ohio State University 1948
	B.S. degree on Pharmacy, Ohio State University 1951
Military Service:	None
Pharmacy Practice:	Staff Pharmacist, J.H. Beam Drug Company 1954 – 1965
	Owner, Buch and Donovan Drugstore, Wheeling 1965 – 2002
Notable Facts:	President, Ohio-Marshall Counties Pharmacy Association
	President, Moundsville Rotary International

Name:	*Everett Burton "Bud" Stanley,* Seventy-Second President
Birth/Death:	1928 – 2003
Education:	B.S., WVU College of Pharmacy 1952
Military Service:	None
Pharmacy Practice:	Owner, Town and Country, Nutter Fort, WV 1964 – 1979
	Bland's Drug Store, Clarksburg, WV 1979 – 1979

Name:	*Robert William Johnson,* Seventy-Third President
Birth/Death:	1926 – 1984
Education:	B.S. Pharmacy, University of Iowa College of Pharmacy 1950
Military Service:	U.S. Army * in FECOM during World War II
Pharmacy Practice:	Pharmacist, White Cross Pharmacy, Huntington, WV 1957 – 1976
	Veterans Administration Hospital 1976 – 1984

Notable Facts:	Member, WVPA
	Served in every office of SWVPA
	Board of Directors, SWVPA
	Clinical Instructor, WVU School of Pharmacy

*Robert, who enlisted at age seventeen, served with the 383rd Infantry Regiment, 96th Infantry Division, where — as a squad leader — he fought in the Philippines and Okinawa, and was wounded both on Leyte and Okinawa. Robert was a recipient of a Bronze Star medal and the Purple Heart with Oak Leaf Cluster.

Name:	*Edward Arthur Toompas,* Seventy-Fourth President	
Birth/Death:	1952 – 1994	
Education:	B.S., WVU School of Pharmacy	1952
Military Service:	U.S. Army, Ft. Benning, GA	1952 – 1955
Pharmacy Practice:	Bland's Drug Store, Clarksburg, WV	1955 – 1993

Name:	*James Keith Coleman,* Seventy-Fifth President	
Birth/Death:	1942 –	
Education:	B.S., WVU School of Pharmacy	1965
Military Service:	None	
Pharmacy Practice:	Staff Pharmacist, Watkins Drug Co., Beckley, WV	1965
	Owner, Coleman's Pharmacy	1966 – 1976
	Monroe Pharmacy	
	Owner, Alderson Pharmacy	1973 – Present
Notable Facts:	Past President WVPA	1981
	Grand High Priest, Royal Arch Masons of WV	
	Grand Commander, Knights Templer of WV	

Name:	*Scot Alan Anderson,* Seventy-Sixth President	
Birth/Death:	1945 –	
Education:	B.S., WVU School of Pharmacy	1968
Military Service:	None	
Pharmacy Practice:	Fredlock's Pharmacy, Morgantown, WV	1968 – 1975
	Owner, Suncrest Pharmacy, Morgantown, WV	1975 – Present
Notable Facts:	President, WVPA	1982 – 1983
	President, Mon Valley Pharmacists Association	Unknown
	Treasurer, WVPA	1978 – 1981
	President, WVU School of Pharmacy Alumni Association	1994 – 1995
	Member, Tripartite Committee for WVU Student Clinical Rotations	

Name:	*Arlie Arnold Winters,* Seventy-Seventh President	
Birth/Death:	1932 –	
Education:	B.S., WVU College of Pharmacy	1954
	Eastern Kentucky University National Certified Inspector/Investigator Training Program	1997
Military Service:	Pharmacy Officer, 98th General Hospital, Neubrucke, Germany	1957 – 1959
Pharmacy Practice:	Morrison's Drug Store, Terra Alta, WV	1953 – 1954
	Pharmacist, Whelan Drug Store, Morgantown	1954 – 1957
	Pharmacist, Malone's Drug Store, Grafton, WV	1955 – 1957
	First Lieutenant, MSC, U.S. Army (Res)	1957
	Owner, Community Pharmacy, Berkeley Springs, WV	1959 – 1985
	Staff Pharmacist, War Memorial Hospital	1959 – 1982
	Staff Pharmacist, Kings Daughters Hospital	1960 – 1962
	Consultant, Valley View Nursing Home	1972 – 1984
	Inspector, WV Board of Pharmacy	1986 – Present

Notable Facts:	President, WVPA	1983 – 1984
	President, WVU School of Pharmacy Alumni	
	Association	1966 – 1967
	President, Eastern WV Academy of Pharmacy	1966 – 1967
	Member, Morgan County Board of Education	1972 – 1978
	Member, Council, Town of Bath	1984 – 1985
	Recipient, Outstanding Service to the WVU	
	School of Pharmacy Award	1979
	Recipient, Dr. James Hartley Beal Award	1991

Name:	*Frank J. McClendon*, Seventy-Eighth President	
Birth/Death:	1953 –	
Education:	B.S., WVU School of Pharmacy	1977
Pharmacy Practice:	Pharmacist, Highlawn Pharmacy,	
	Huntington, WV	1977 – 1985
	President & CEO, Creative Professional	
	Marketing	1980 – 1987
	COO/PIC/Owner, Comprecare (Option Care)	1985 – Present
Notable Facts:	President, WVPA	1984 – 1985
	Co-Author of a Pharmacy Text Book, *Sexual*	
	Health, published by Simon and Schuster	1984
	Recipient, WVPA Board of Directors Award	1979
	Recipient, NARD Pharmacy Leadership Award	1984
	Recipient, WVPA Presidents Award	1985

Name:	*Thomas Edward Menighan*, Seventy-Ninth President	
Birth/Death:	1952 –	
Education:	B.S. cum laude in Pharmacy, WVU School of Pharmacy	1974
	MBA, Averett College	1990
Pharmacy Practice:	Chain Store Pharmacist, Zanesville, Ohio	1974 – 1976
	Manager, Chain Pharmacy, Danville, Virginia	1976 – 1978
	Owner, Medicine Shoppe Pharmacy, Huntington	1978 – 1998
	Founded Option Care Home Infusion Services	1981
	Vice President for Operations, Pharmark Corp	1992 – 1993
	President & CEO, SymRx, Inc., Rockville, MD	2000 – 2005
	Currently, President of SynTegra, LLC	2005 – Present
Notable Facts:	Recipient, Bowl of Hygeia Award	1984

Recipient, NARD Pharmacy Leadership Award		1985
Recipient, WVU School of Pharmacy Preceptor of the Year Award		1986
Recipient, WVU School of Pharmacy Outstanding Alumnus Award		1987
Recipient, Merck Outstanding Achievement Award		1995
Recipient, Dr. James Hartley Beal Award		1999

Name: *Sandra Elizabeth Justice,* Eightieth President of WVPA

Birth/Death: 1954 –

Education: B.S., WVU School of Pharmacy   1978

Military Service: None

Pharmacy Practice: Community Pharmacy Practice, Montgomery, WV   1978 – 1995

Pharmaceutical Consulting: (Managed WV Medicaid Retro Drug Utilization Review Program)   1995 – 1999

DUR Program Management/Development of Continuing Education Programs   1999 – 2004

President, Kanawha Valley Pharmacists Association   1986 – 1994

President, WVPA   1986 – 1987

Board of Trustees, APhA   1994 – 1997

Member, WV State Board of Pharmacy   1989 – 1995

Chair, DUR Committee, WV Department HHS   1991 – 1995

President, WVU School of Pharmacy Alumni Association   1989 – 1990

Owner, Nora Apothecary, Indianapolis, IN   1996 – Present

Notable Facts: Recipient, NARD Pharmacy Leadership Award   1986

Recipient, Squibb Presidents Award   1987

Kanawha Valley Pharmacists Association Leadership Award   1985

Recipient, WVPA Presidents Award   1989, 1992, 1994

Phi Lambda Sigma National Leadership Honorary   1991

Recipient, WV School of Pharmacy Outstanding Service Award   1991

Recipient, Bowl of Hygeia Award   1991

Recipient, Dr. James Hartley Beal Award   1997

Name:	*Robert Neil Lohr,* Eighty-First President	
Birth/Death:	1950 –	
Education:	B.S., WVU School of Pharmacy	1974
Military Service:	None	

Pharmacy Practice:	Owner, Princeton Pharmacy	1974 – 1996
	Owner, Princeton Pharmacy Institutional	1995 – 1998
	Owner, Bluewell Pharmacy	1974 – 1996
	Pharmacist-in-Charge, SunScript Pharmacy	1998 – 2000
	Consulting Pharmacist, Omnicare	2000 – Present
	Correctional Medical Systems	2000 – Present

Notable Facts:	President, WVPA	1987 – 1988
	Secretary-Treasurer, Southern Appalachian Pharmacists Association, Princeton, WV	1979 – 1984
	President, Southern Appalachian Pharmacists Association, Princeton, WV	1984 – 1986
	William S. Apple Program in Community Pharmacy Management	1988
	Member, WVU School of Pharmacy Visiting Committee	1976 – 1978
	Chair, Princeton Planning Commission	1996 – 2006
	Board of Directors, Rotary International	1975 – 1994
	Recipient, Princeton Rotary Rotarian of the Year	
	President, United Methodist Men, WV Methodist Conference, Princeton, WV	1996 – 2000
	Recipient, The Torch Award, United Methodist Men	
	Recipient, Bowl of Hygeia Award	1983
	Recipient, Dr. James Hartley Beal Award	2003

Name:	*Debra Warden Nichol,* Eighty-Second President	
Birth/Death:	1956 –	
Education:	B.S., WVU School of Pharmacy	1979

Pharmacy Practice:

Staff Pharmacist, Super X Drug Corporation, Beckley, WV	1979 – 1984
Director, Pharmacy Services, New River Family Health Center, Scarbro, WV	1984 – 1989
Director of Professional Affairs, WVPA	1989 – 1991
Owner, South Park Pharmacy, Coral Gables, FL	1991 – 1995
Director of Professional/Educational Affairs, New Jersey Pharmacists Association, Trenton, NJ	1995 – 1998
Staff Pharmacist, CVS, Beckley, WV	1998 – 1999
Staff Pharmacist, Raleigh General Hospital, Beckley, WV	1999 – 2001
Director, Pharmacy Services, Beckley Health Right Clinic, Beckley, WV	2001 – 2004
Pharmacist, Walmart Pharmacy, Beckley, WV	2004 – Present

Notable Facts:

President, WVPA	1988 – 1989
Chair, Administrative Practice Section, Academy of Pharmacy Practice Pharmacy Practice and Management, APhA	1991 – 1993
Member, Executive Committee, Florida Pharmacists Association	1992 – 1993
President, Dade County Florida Pharmacists Association	1992 – 1993
President, Board of Directors, WVPA Recovery Network	2004 – Present
Recipient, NCPA Leadership Award, WVPA	1988
Recipient, Squibb Pharmacy Leadership Award	1989
Recipient, Merck Award, Dade County Florida Pharmacists Association	1992
Recipient, APhA Most Innovative Pharmacy Practice Award	1993
Recipient, APhA Academy Pharmacy Practice Management Award	1993

Name:	*Robert Joseph Coram,* Eighty-Third President	
Birth/Death:	1956 –	
Education:	B.S., WVU School of Pharmacy	1979
	M.S. in Business Administration, WVU College of Business and Economics	1992
Military Service:	None	
Pharmacy Practice:	Pharmacist, Medical Center Hospital Chillicothe, Ohio	1979 – 1980
	Pharmacist, Ohio Valley Hospital, Steubenville, Ohio	1980 – 1980
	Pharmacist, Wheeling Hospital, Wheeling, WV	1980 – 1986
	Director of Pharmacy, Wheeling Hospital	1986 – 2006
Notable Facts:	President, Ohio-Marshall County Pharmacists Association	1983 – 1984
	President, WV Society of Health System Pharmacists	1988 – 1989
	President, WVPA	1989 – 1990
	President, WVU School of Pharmacy Alumni Association	1999 – 2000
	Recipient, NARD Pharmacy Leadership Award	1989
	Recipient, Squibb Pharmacy Leadership Award	1990
	Recipient, Ohio-Marshall County Pharmacists Association Pharmacist of the Year Award	1993

Name:	*Charles Vinton Selby, Jr.,* Eighty-Fourth President	
Birth/Death:	1938 –	
Education:	B.S., WVU School of Pharmacy	1962
Military Service:	United States Navy, Officers Candidate School	1962
	Line Officer, U.S.N., USS Falgout DER 324	1962 – 1964
Pharmacy Practice:	Staff Pharmacist, Selby Drug Company, Clarksburg, WV	1964 – 1967
	Pharmacist-in-Charge, Staats Drug Store, Spencer, WV	1967 – 1971
	Pharmacist-in-Charge, Appalachian Regional Hospital, Beckley, WV	1971 – 1975

	Staff Pharmacist, Medical Arts Pharmacy, Beckley, WV	1976 – 1978
	Pharmacist-in-Charge, Carriage Drive Pharmacy, Beckley, WV	1979 – 1986
	Director of Pharmacy, Community Health Systems, Beckley, WV	1987 – 1999
	Pharmacist, Veterans Administration Medical Center, Beckley, WV	1999 – Present
Notable Facts:	President, WVPA	1990 – 1991
	Treasurer, WVPA	1995 – 1997
	Secretary-Treasurer, New River Pharmacists Association	1972 – 1997
	Recipient, Bowl of Hygeia Award	1992
	Treasurer, American College of Apothecaries	1958 – 1960

Name:	*Marvin Todd Way,* Eighty-Fifth President	
Birth/Death:	1959 –	
Education:	B.S., WVU School of Pharmacy	1983
Military Service:	None	
Pharmacy Practice:	Vice President, Valley Health	
Notable Facts:	President, WVPA	1991 – 1992
	President, West Virginia Society of Hospital Pharmacists	1995 – 1996
	Recipient, Distinguished Young Pharmacist Award	1991

Name:	*Karen Lynn Reed,* Eighty-Sixth President	
Birth/Death:	1957 –	
Education:	B.S., WVU School of Pharmacy	1980
	Disease State Management Certificate Program	1996
Military Service:	None	
Pharmacy Practice:	Pharmacist, Kmart Pharmacy, Beckley, WV	2002 – Present
	Consultant Pharmacist, Beckley Surgery Center	1999 – Present
	Owner, Contact Pharmacy, Beckley, WV	1986 – 2001
	Staff Pharmacist, Appalachian Regional Hospital, Beckley, WV	1980 – 1984

Notable Facts:	President, WVPA	1992 – 1993
	President, New River Pharmaceutical Association	1986 – 1988
	President, WVU School of Pharmacy Alumni Association	1998 – 1999
	Member, APhA Board of Trustees	2003 – 2006
	Recipient, WVPA Presidents Award	1989
	Recipient, Marion Merrell Dow Distinguished Young Pharmacist Award	1989
	Recipient, NARD Pharmacy Leadership Award	1992
	Recipient, Bristol Myers Squibb Pharmacy Leadership Award	1993
	Recipient, Bowl of Hygeia Award	1995
	Recipient, Merck Pharmacy Achievement Award	1997
	Fellow, APhA	2000

Name:	*Roger Scott Cole,* Eighty-Seventh President	
Birth/Death:	1953 –	
Education:	B.S., WVU School of Pharmacy	1976
Military Service:	None	
Pharmacy Practice:	Owner, Medicine Shoppe Pharmacy	1981 – 2000
	Owner, Moundsville Pharmacy	2000 – Present
Notable Facts:	President, WVPA	1993 – 1994
	Two term president, Ohio- Marshall County Pharmacists Association	1982 – 1983, 1987 – 1988
	Recipient, NARD Leadership Award	1993
	Recipient, McKesson Leadership Award	1994
	Recipient, Bowl of Hygeia Award	1999
	Recipient (twice), Ohio - Marshall Counties Pharmacist of the Year Award	1991, 1999

Name:	*Zachariah Taylor Phillips III,* Eighty-Eighth President	
Birth/Death:	1952 –	
Education:	B.S., WVU School of Pharmacy	1975
Military Service:	None	

Pharmacy Practice:	Staff Pharmacist, Thrift Drug, Bluefield, WV	1975 – 1978
	Staff Pharmacist, CVS Pharmacy, Sophia, WV	1978 – present
Notable Facts:	Secretary, WVPA	1992 – 1994
	President, WVPA	1994 – 1995
	President, New River Pharmacists Association	1986 – 1988

Name: *Carol Ann Hudachek,* Eighty-Ninth President

Birth/Death: 1952 –

Education:	B.A., Biology, West Virginia University	1973
	M.A., Secondary Education, WVU	1977
	B.S., WVU School of Pharmacy	1987
	Pharm.D., WVU School of Pharmacy	2003

Military Service: None

Pharmacy Practice:	Clinical Pharmacist, Weirton Medical Center	1987 – 2002
	Clinical Pharmacy Manager, Cardinal Health	2003 – 2006
Notable Facts:	Recipient, Marion-Merrill Dow Distinguished	
	Young Pharmacist Award	1990
	President, WVPA	1994 – 1995
	President, WV Society Health Systems	
	Pharmacists	1997 – 1999
	Recipient, NARD Leadership Award	1995
	Recipient, Merck Community Service Award	1998
	Recipient, Ohio-Marshall County Pharmacist	
	of the Year Award	1998
	Recipient, Bowl of Hygeia Award	2004

Name: *Steven Craig Judy,* Ninetieth President

Birth/Death: 1952 –

| **Education:** | B.S., WVU School of Pharmacy | 1975 |

Military Service: None

| **Pharmacy Practice:** | Clinical Rural Pharmacy Practice, | |
| | Petersburg, WV | 1975 – 2006 |

Notable Facts:	Chair, Grant County Board of Health	1987 – 2006
	Member, Grant County Chamber of Commerce	
	Director, Highland Bank Shares	2000 – 2006
	Director, Grant County Bank	1992 – 2006
	President, WVPA	1996 – 1997
	Member, West Virginia Board of Pharmacy	2000 – 2004
	Recipient, Dr. James Hartley Beal Award	2001
	President, WVU School of Pharmacy Alumni Association	2004 – 2005
	Recipient, Bowl of Hygeia Award	2005

Name:	*William S. McFarland,* Ninety-First President	
Birth/Death:	1947 –	
Education:	WVU undergraduate general studies	1965 – 1967
	B.S., Pharmacy, University of Texas, Austin	1972
Military Service:	U.S. Army (Viet Nam)	1967 – 1970
Highest Rank Held:	Sergeant	
Pharmacy Practice:	Staff Pharmacist, St. Albans, WV	1972 – 1973
	Staff Pharmacist, St. Albans Super X pharmacy	1973 – 1974
	Staff Pharmacist, St. Albans Rite Aid pharmacy	1974 – 1982
	Staff Pharmacist, Kanawha Valley Hospital	1982 – 1984
	Owner, Loop Plaza Pharmacy, St. Albans, WV	1984 – Present
Notable Facts:	Recipient, Bowl of Hygeia Award	2001

Name:	*John Joseph Bernabei,* Ninety-Second President	
Birth/Death:	1966	
Education:	B.S., WVU School of Pharmacy	1988
Military Service:	None	
Pharmacy Practice:	Staff Pharmacist, Rite Aid Pharmacy, Parsons, WV	1988 – 1990
	Staff Pharmacist, Hood's Pharmacy, Follonsbee, WV	1990 – 1994
	Staff Pharmacist, Weirton Medical Center Pharmacy, Weirton, WV	1994 – 1996
	Staff Pharmacist, Tri-State Medical Group, Weirton, WV	1996 – Present

Notable Facts:	President, WVPA	1997 – 1998
	Member, Board of Directors, Weirton Area	
	Salvation Army	
	Member, Board of Directors, Weirton Area	
	Chamber of Commerce	
	Member, Board of Advisors, CHANGE	

Name:	*Maribeth Bee Nobles,* Ninety-Third President	
Birth/Death:	1966 –	
Education:	B.S. (cum laude) in Marine Biology, University of North Carolina	1988
	B.S., WVU School of Pharmacy	1990
Military Service:	None	
Pharmacy Practice:	Staff Pharmacist, Veterans Administration Medical Center, Martinsburg, WV	1998 – Present
	Manager, Martin's Pharmacy, Charles Town, WV	1998 – 1998
	Staff Pharmacist, CVS Pharmacy, Martinsburg, WV	1997 – 1998
	Manager, Patterson's Drug Store, Martinsburg, WV	1996 – 1997
	Manager, Kroger Pharmacy, Cross Lanes, WV	1992 – 1996
	Manager, Rite Aid Pharmacy, South Charleston, WV	1991 – 1992
Notable Facts:	President, WVPA	1999 – 2000
	Member, Board of Directors, WVPA	1997 – 1998
	Recipient, DuPont Innovative Pharmacy Practice Award	1994
	Recipient, Marion Merrill Dow Distinguished Young Pharmacist Award	1994
	Recipient, Bristol-Myers Squibb Pharmacy Leadership Award	1999
	Recipient, NARD Pharmacy Leadership Award	1999
	Recipient, Merck Pharmacist Achievement Award	2000

Name:	*Joseph Craig McGlothlin,* Ninety-Fourth President	
Birth/Death:	1956 –	
Education:	B.S. (magma cum laude), WVU School of Pharmacy	1981
Military Service:	None	
Pharmacy Practice:	Staff Pharmacist, SuperRx, Bluefield, WV	1981 – 1984
	Kings Daughters Hospital, Ashland, KY	1985 – 1986
	Staff Pharmacist, SuperRx, Ashland, KY	1986
	Owner, Medicine Shoppe, Huntington	1987 – Present
Notable Facts:	President, WVPA	1999 – 2000
	Member of Board, United Methodist Church, Kenova, WV	2004 – Present
	Recipient, National Community Pharmacists Association Pharmacy Leadership Award	2001
	Recipient, Merck Pharmacists Achievement Award	2001

Name:	*Carl Joseph Malanga,* Ninety-Fifth President	
Birth/Death:	1939 –	
Education:	B.S. (magna cum laude), Fordham University College of Pharmacy	1961
	M.S., Department of Biological Sciences, Fordham University	1967
	Ph.D., Department of Biological Sciences, Fordham University	1970
Military Service:	U.S. Army, First Lieutenant, Infantry	1962 – 1964
Pharmacy Practice:	Community Pharmacy Practice (New York State)	1964 – 1970
Notable Facts:	Associate Dean, WVU School of Pharmacy	1991 – 2002
	Faculty Advisor, WVU Pharmacy Honors Program	1991 – 2002
	Faculty Advisor for all Pre-Pharmacy Students	1991 – 2002
	Recipient, Borden Outstanding Freshman Prize	1958
	Recipient, Merck Award	1961
	Recipient, Bristol Award	1961
	Valedictorian, Class of 1961	

President, Rho Chi Honor Society, Beta Xi Chapter	1960
Sigma Xi	1972
Outstanding Educators of America	1972
Recipient, Thirteen WVU School of Pharmacy Outstanding Teacher Awards	1974 – 1997
WVU Foundation Award for Outstanding Teaching	1994
Golden Key Honor Society, Golden Apple Award	1995
President, WVPA	2001 – 2002
Emeritus Professor of Pharmacy	2002 – Present

Name:	*John Ervin Corkrean,* Ninety-Sixth President	
Birth/Death:	1951 –	
Education:	B.S., WVU School of Pharmacy	1974
Pharmacy Practice:	Pharmacist, Ralston's Drug Store, Weston, WV	1974 – 1978
	Pharmacist/owner, Staats Pharmacy, Spencer, WV	1978 – Present
Notable Facts:	Member, Spencer City Council	1985 – 1987
	Director, Roane County Chamber of Commerce	1997 – Present
	President, WVPA	2002 – 2003
	Member, Board of Directors, WVPA	2003 – 2004
	Recipient, Bowl of Hygeia Award	1996

Name:	*Patty Carol Johnston,* Ninety-Seventh President	
Birth/Death:	1954 –	
Education:	B.S. (cum laude), WVU School of Pharmacy	1977
Military Service:	None	
Pharmacy Practice:	Staff Pharmacist, Medical Arts Pharmacy	1977 – 1978
	Staff Pharmacist/Nursing Home Consultant, Doctors Clinic Pharmacy	1978 – 1986
	Owner, Colony Drug and Wellness Center	1986 – Present

Notable Facts:	President, WVPA	2003 – 2004
	President-elect, WVPA	2002 – 2003
	President, New River Pharmacists Association	1980 – 1981
	Recipient, Dr. James Hartley Beal Award	2005
	WV Cost Management Council (Est. by the WV State Legislature)	2004 –
	Board of Advisors, WVU School of Pharmacy	1979 – 1981
		2004 – Present
	Ernst & Young Entrepreneur of the Year Award	2003
	Preceptor of the Year Award, WVU School of Pharmacy	2001
	WVPA's Elan Pharmaceutical Innovative Practice Award	2002
	WVU School of Pharmacy Alumni Advisory Council	2000 – Present
	President, Beckley Civitan Club	1991 – 1992
	Member, Beckley-Raleigh County Chamber of Commerce	1986 – Present
	Member, WV Medicaid Retro DUR Committee	1994 – 1998

Name:	*Eric Michael Lambert,* Ninety-Eighth President	
Birth/Death:	1969 –	
Education:	B.S., WVU School of Pharmacy	1993
Military Service:	None	
Pharmacy Practice:	Staff Pharmacist, Fruth Pharmacy	1994 – 1999
	Fruth Pharmacy: Director of Pharmacy	1999 – Present
Notable Facts:	Recipient, Distinguished Young Pharmacists Award	2002
	Recipient, National Community Pharmacists Association Leadership Award	2004
	Recipient, National Community Pharmacists Association - Bristol Myers Corporation Leadership Award	2005
	Recipient, Merck Pharmacists Achievement Award	2005

Name:	*Dennis Ray Lewis,* Ninety-Ninth President	
Birth/Death:	1952 –	
Education:	B.S. in Mathematics, Concord College, Athens, WV	1974
	B.S. (cum laude), WVU School of Pharmacy	1977
	Ordained as Baptist minister	2004
Military Service:	None	
Pharmacy Practice:	Staff Pharmacist, Rite Aid Pharmacy	1977 – 1980
	Founder/Vice President, Durable Technical, Inc	1981 – 1984
	Founder/President, Health Care Pharmacy, Inc.	1984 – 1998
	Harwood and Lewis Associated, Inc., (Real Estate)	1983 – Present
	Nursing Home Care, Inc.	1996 – 1998
	Founder, Dignity Hospice of Southern WV, Chapmanville, WV	1993 – Present
	First Healthcare Associates, Inc.	1996 – 1998
Notable Facts:	President, WVPA	2005 – 2006
	Recipient, Merck Community Service Award	2005
	Recipient, DuPont Innovative Pharmacists Practice Award	1995
	Recipient, Ernest & Young Entrepreneur of the Year Award	1993
Community Service:	President, Dignity Hospice of Southern WV	
	Director, West Virginia Baptist Foundation	
	Member of Board, Logan - Mingo Area Mental Health, Inc.	

Name:	*Keith Andrew Foster,* One-Hundredth President	
Birth/Death:	1961 –	
Education:	B.S., WVU School of Pharmacy	1984
	National Certification, Pharmacy Based Immunization Delivery	2006
	Certified, Pharmacy Based Self-Care Services	2004
	Certified, Anticoagulation Therapy	1999
	Pharmaceutical Care for patients with diabetes	2004
	Certified, Menopause Management	2000

Military Service:	None	
Pharmacy Practice:	Staff Pharmacist, Revco Pharmacy, Winchester VA	1984 – 1985
	Staff Pharmacist, Revco Pharmacy, Beckley, WV	1985 – 1997
	Staff Pharmacist, Colony Drug and Wellness Center, Beckley, WV	1997 – Present
Notable Facts:	Member, New River Pharmacists Association	1990 – Present
	Adjunct Clinical Instructor, WVU School of Pharmacy	1995 – Present
	Fellow, American College of Apothecaries	2000 – Present
	Member, American Association of Diabetes Educators	2004 – Present
	Member, American Diabetes Association	2004 – Present
	President, WVPA	2006 – 2007

Name:	*David Earl Flynn,* One Hundred First President	
Birth/Death:	1957 –	
Education:	Associate Degree in Science, Community College, Allegheny County (PA)	1978
	B.S. (cum laude) in Pharmacy, University of Pittsburgh School of Pharmacy	1983
Military Service:	None	
Pharmacy Practice:	Manager, Rite Aid Pharmacy, Clay, WV	1983 – 1985
	Supervisor, Rite Aid Pharmacy, North Central West Virginia	1985 – 1995
	Rite Aid Pharmacy Development Manager,	1995 – 2002
	WVU Hospital Pharmacy, Morgantown, WV	2002 – Present
Notable Facts:	Adjunct Assistant Professor, WVU School of Pharmacy,	1990 – Present
	Board Member, Monongalia County Mass Transit Authority,	2002 – Present
	Board Member, Milan Puskar Health Right Clinic	2004 – Present
	WVU School of Pharmacy Continuing Education Committee	2003 – Present
	WVU Hospital Safety Committee	2005 – Present

First grade teacher AWANA club at
    Faith Baptist Church   2005 – Present
Recipient, Rite Aid Eastern Divisional Pharmacy
    Supervisor of the year Award   1994
Recipient, Rite Aid Pharmacy Development
    Manager Award   1997
Recipient, Rite Aid Pharmacy Development
    Manager Award   2000
Recipient, ASHP Courageous Service Award   2006
Recipient, NCPA Leadership Award   2008

Appendix F

Distinguished Young Pharmacist Award
Honor Roll of Recipients

Year	Name	Home
1987	J. Douglas Hammond	Elkins
1988	Jeanette C. Smith	Beckley
1989	Karen L. Reed	Beckley
1990	Carol Ann Hudachek	Weirton
1991	M. Todd Way	Martinsburg
1992	Robert Kelly Massie, Jr.	Princeton
1993	Lance Everett Rhodes	Nitro
1994	Maribeth Bee Nobles	Dunbar
1995	Jann Burks Hinkle	Falls Church, VA
1996	Shannon Stanley	Charleston
1997	Amy Wayne Brabbin	Charleston
1998	No Nominee	
1999	Lora Lewellyn	St. Albans
2000	Kenneth Reed	Berkeley Springs
2001	No Nominee	
2002	Eric Lambert	Ona
2003	Erin Rudge	St. Albans
2004	Emily Judy	Petersburg
2005	Charles (C.K.) Babcock	Tornado
2006	Betsy Elswick	Morgantown
2007	No Nominee	
2008	Jason M. Turner	Moundsville

Innovative Pharmacy Practice Award
Honor Roll of Recipients

Year	Name	Home
1994	Maribeth Nobles	Dunbar
1994	Shannon Stanley	Charleston
1995	Dennis R. Lewis	Chapmanville
1996	Carol Hudachek	Weirton
1997	Amy Wayne Brabbin	Charleston
1998	No Nominee	
1999	Lora Lewellyn	St. Albans
2000	Barbara D. Smith	Spencer
2001	Sue and J. J. Bernabei	Follansbee
2002	Patricia C. Johnston	Beckley
2003	William S. McFarland	St. Albans
2004	No Nominee	
2005	Betsy Meredith Elswick	Morgantown

Dr. James Hartley Beal Award
Honor Roll of Recipients

Year	Name	Home
1947	J. Lester Hayman	Morgantown
1949	Roy Bird Cook	Charleston
1951	George Orville Young	Buckhannon
1953	Ernest K. Hoge	Wheeling
1955	Fred C. Allen	Marlinton
1957	Gordon Alger Bergy	Morgantown
1961	William J. Dixon	Oak Hill
1963	Clyde N. Roberts	Huntington
1965	Edgar B. Moore	Clarksburg
1967	Charles Herbert Traubert	Follansbee
1969	Albert Flurnoy Bond	Clendenin
1971	Frederick Linck Geiler	Morgantown
1973	William B. Stuck	Charleston
1975	William Sidney Coleman	Lewisburg
1977	Virgil R. Hertzog	Worthington
1979	Guy N. Lang	Moorefield
1981	Albert Freddie Wojcik	Morgantown
1983	David Stephen Crawford	Elkins
1987	John Patrick Plummer	Fairmont
1989	Douglas Dennis Glover	Morgantown
1991	Arlie Arnold Winters, Jr.	Berkeley Springs
1993	Thomas H. Carson	Montgomery
1995	Jack Edward Fruth	Point Pleasant
1997	Sandra Elizabeth Justice	Charleston
1999	Thomas E. Menighan	Huntington
2001	Steve C. Judy	Petersburg
2003	Robert N. Lohr	Princeton
2005	Patricia Johnston	Beckley
2007	Roger Cole	Moundsville

Bowl of Hygeia Award
Honor Roll of Recipients

Year	Name	Home
1959	Charles Horner Troxell	Fairmont
1960	Joseph W. Pugh	Martinsburg
1961	Minter B. Ralston	Weston
1962	Guy N. Lang	Moorefield
1963	Ann Dinardi	Morgantown
1964	Edward B. Moore	Clarksburg
1965	Stephen B. Thompson	Vienna
1966	William Sidney Coleman	Lewisburg
1967	Joseph G. Stevens	Huntington
1968	Francis B. Wimmer	Princeton
1969	Isadore R. Wein	Beckley
1970	Norman S. Bovenizer, Sr.	Bluefield
1971	William J. Plyburn	Barboursville
1972	Claude M. Hamlett	Keystone
1973	Robert H. Shirley	Beckley
1974	Carl E. Furbee, Jr.	Bridgeport
1975	Virgil R. Hertzog	Worthington
1976	William Spencer Coleman	Lewisburg
1977	Jack Edward Fruth	Pt. Pleasant
1978	Maurice Neil Lohr	Princeton
1979	John H. Rice	Shinnston
1980	George E. Fisher, Jr.	Bluefield
1981	Joseph Monti, Jr.	Welch
1982	Sam Kapourales	Williamson
1983	Robert N. Lohr	Princeton

Bowl of Hygeia Award
Honor Roll of Recipients *(Cont'd)*

Year	Name	Home
1984	Thomas Edward Menighan	Huntington
1985	Roger Allen Shallis	Martinsburg
1986	George Karos	Martinsburg
1987	David Stephen Crawford	Elkins
1988	Ernest W. Turner	Huntington
1989	R. Scott Criss	Elkins
1990	David W. Miller	Sistersville
1991	Sandra Elizabeth Justice	Charleston
1992	Charles V. Selby	Beckley
1993	Thomas L. Carson	Montgomery
1994	Donley W. Hutson	Nutter Fort
1995	Karen L. Reed	Beckley
1996	John E. Corkrean	Spencer
1997	Gary Mastromichales	Weirton
1998	Richard Griffin	Kenova
1999	Roger S. Coleman, Sr.	Wheeling
2000	Carol Ann Hudachek	Weirton
2001	William McFarland	St. Albans
2002	Lydia DeBoni Main	Masontown
2003	Lora Lewellyn Good	Elkview
2004	Charles Burdette	Milton
2005	Steve Judy	Petersburg
2006	John J. Bernabei	Weirton
2007	Kelly Massie	Beckley
2008	Susan P. Meredith	Shinnston

Photographs

Chapter	Subject	Source of Photograph
Chapter 1	Dr. James Hartley Beal	Gregory Higby, American Institute of History of Pharmacy, Madison, WI
	Gordon A. Bergy	WVU School of Pharmacy
	Figure 1	WVU School of Pharmacy
Chapter 2	Cascarets advertisement	Betty Jean Wymer, Oglebay Institute, Wheeling, WV
	William E. Weiss	Betty Jean Wymer, Oglebay Institute, Wheeling, WV
Chapter 3	Lydia Main	WVU School of Pharmacy
	Donald Sinclair	Mrs. D.C. Sinclair
	Carl E. Furbee	*West Virginia Pharmacist*
	William Plyburn	Jim Plyburn
	James L. Turner	John Veasey
	William S. Coleman	*West Virginia Pharmacist*
	Sam Kapourales	*West Virginia Pharmacist*
	Charles Blissitt	City of Morgantown
Chapter 4	Senator Fred C. Allen	*West Virginia Pharmacist*
	Senator G. O. Young	*West Virginia Pharmacist*
	Senator Herbert Traubert	*West Virginia Pharmacist*
	Gov. Okey Patteson	West Virginia University Publication Services
Chapter 5	S/Sgt Ralph Stevenson	Ralph Stevenson
	Brig. General Jack Halki	Betsy Halki
	John P. Plummer	WVU School of Pharmacy
	Major Michael A. Rafferty	*Charleston (WV) Gazette*
	Lt. Rockis in Korea	Vickie Rockis
	Fredlock & Zimmerman on Pork Chop Hill	Douglas Glover
	Lt. Glover in Korea	Douglas Glover

About the Author

Douglas Glover is a native West Virginian whose father practiced pharmacy in a small rural community in northern West Virginia. As a youth, he worked in his father's drug store, performing such duties as janitor, tending the soda fountain, and home delivery of medications. Enrolling in the West Virginia University College of Pharmacy, he graduated with the class of 1951 and served in the U.S. Army in Korea. After the war, he practiced pharmacy in West Virginia for four years before entering Emory University School of Medicine. An obstetrics and gynecology residency at Grady Memorial Hospital in Atlanta was followed by a seventeen-year practice of medicine in Marietta, Georgia. Returning to West Virginia in 1982, he entered academic medicine and taught medical students in a series of clinics in underserved rural communities in southern West Virginia and adjacent counties of Ohio.

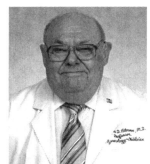

Douglas Glover

Recruited to West Virginia University in 1987 with a joint appointment as professor of obstetrics and gynecology in the School of Medicine and clinical professor of pharmacy in the School of Pharmacy, Glover established five rural outreach clinics in which he taught medical and pharmacy students. His research in medication use in pregnancy and pharmacokinetics of drugs in the pregnant woman has been published in forty-three scientific papers in peer-reviewed journals and nineteen book chapters. He was previously Associate Editor of a textbook, *Current Therapy in Obstetrics.*

Retiring from medical practice, Glover spent four years researching this book and conducted interviews of one hundred sixty-five pharmacists for their stories.

Author photo by Bob Beverly

2615159

Made in the USA